VACCINATION
I$ NOT
IMMUNIZATION

second edition

_____Dr. Tim O'Shea _____

copyright MMXII   immunition ltd

vaccination is not immunization 2nd edition / Tim O'Shea

Library of Congress   Cataloguing-in-Publications
99-95690

ISBN: 1-929487-13-4

Cover design: Eric Phan

immunition ltd
915.307.1055
www.thedoctorwithin.com

Printed in the United States of America

It is impossible to estimate the true value of Dr O'Shea's work. His review of the history of the vaccination industry is vastly more thorough than that taught in medical schools and decisively more balanced.

Many primary care providers and parents who assume that the vaccine program was built on sound principles will be shocked at the flimsy foundations of immunization science. More relevant than its roots, what every parent and doctor must decide is whether the risks of vaccination are offset by the potential benefits. While the public is rarely exposed to the full extent of vaccine adverse reactions, Dr O'Shea takes the reader through a thorough review of each "vaccine-preventable" disease and the risk/benefit of their vaccine counterpart.

The book will serve as a valuable resource to parents and physicians who wish to gain further knowledge and understanding of the risk and benefits of the numerous shots being promoted for the proclaimed benefit of public health. Parents need no longer feel guilty or confused about the decision to vaccinate their children. Knowledge is the freedom and power to decide with confidence what is best for their children.

With explosions in chronic illnesses in virtually all subsets of our population, critical thinking is necessary to protect our loved ones and our future. Dr O'Shea has once again blessed us with an up-to-date resource that will allow parents to make an informed choice, and for medical professionals to take pause at what they had been indoctrinated to believe was valid science and good medicine.

David Ayoub, MD
Clinical Radiologist
Springfield, Illinois

Foreword

Whether or not to vaccinate is the most important decision a parent will make in the child's entire life. Nothing is more delicate than the infant brain and the infant immune system, as they struggle into existence. Vaccines have the undisputed ability to damage both.

This book is a meticulously referenced summary of the best, most reliable sources which call into question our vaccine policies. As you will see, opposition to vaccines today is coming not primarily from the holistic arena, but rather from mainstream science, medicine, and law. This book draws from that data.

Mark Twain said that when we buy a book we are pretending to be buying the time to read it. This book can be read in a day or so. But most who get the book never read it, except maybe for a few minutes of skimming. Don't be in that group. If you've always suspected there may be something wrong with vaccines that your doctor and the evening newsreaders might not be telling you, this book will clear all that up. Reading the whole thing can save you months of research, distilling down the key issues. The alternative is blind submission to the unquestioning acquiescence of the flock, consigning your child to the disquieting level of health shared by the majority of children in this country today.

This book is a review of the literature in a field which might be called Problems with Vaccines. It is not a light novel. Speedreading it will certainly sell the reader short. Start at the front cover. Don't stop till you get to the back cover. Only then can responsible parents hope to have an introduction to the effects of vaccines on the fragile and tenuous nature of their infant's formative immune system.

In today's dangerous and toxic world, with so many assaults on human brain neurology, the newborn certainly needs every possible advantage.

Millions of parents learned the score too late: their children are permanently vaccine-damaged. The $2 billion paid out in vaccine injury compensation does not even begin to square the account. And the vast majority of injuries are never reported.

What is the common mantra of those horrified parents? "I wish I'd known" That's what they all say, once they find out, once it's too late.

This is your chance to find out.

Introduction

In this 2nd edition, recent changes in vaccine policy, ignored by most media, are brought to light.

The number of vaccines mandated to US children today follows the exponential rise in global population. In 1974 when world population was at 4 billion, US children were being scheduled for less than 20 vaccines. With world population now at 7 billion, the recommended childhood vaccines in the US have more than tripled, with the current figure at **68**.

Objective investigation finds little scientific justification for this alarming increase. No valid authorities are claiming that the health of American children, by any verifiable index, is anything but appalling – and declining even further. And no matter how they spin it, no one can prove that the increasing number of vaccines has slowed that overall decline one iota.

No child is born with an intact immune system. During the first 2 years of life the immune system is trying desperately to organize. Despite extravagant claims by the medical community, how that immune system is actually assembled by the body is still largely unknown. What is known for certain is that subjecting the infant's immune environment to an array of manmade pathogens, preservatives, and adjuvants absolutely can have a detrimental effect on the formation of that child's brain and nervous system. All scientists – including the vaccine manufacturers – admit as much.

Making one's way through the research in this field, one is continually struck by the endless errors, inconsistency, outright misrepresentation and sheer hubris often found throughout the most prestigious sources of mainstream science, particularly in the publications and FAQs of the CDC, FDA, and NIH. In so many instances it seems clear that their prime objective may not always be presenting the truth, but rather a validation for their own position and power – the eternal *raison d'etre* of the career bureaucrat.

If Nature itself has always gone to extraordinary lengths to protect the blood of the child from outside invasion, can we presume to do any less?

As in the blood, so in the man -
he is just as weak, just as strong.

- Hippocrates

Table of Contents

Money and vaccines	15
History of vaccines: Edward Jenner	17
Smallpox post 9/11	29
Pasteur and the Germ Theory	33
Formaldehyde and aluminum	41
Natural vs. artificial immunity	50
How many vaccinations?	55
The new Adult Schedule	58
Sudden Infant Death Syndrome	60
The Pourcyrous Study	70
Peanut Allergy Epidemic	71
Polio	78
Diphtheria	82
Pertussis	84
Tetanus	86
DPT	91
Shaken Baby	98
Measles	103
Hemophilus influenzae	105
Influenza	108
Swine Flu	112
Hepatitis A	127
Hepatitis B	131
Rotavirus	135
Autism	139
Mercury	142
The death of a child	167
Prevnar	168
Human Papilloma Virus vaccine	172
Doctors who don't vaccinate	184
Exemption Laws	187
Affidavit of Exemption	188
Travel vaccines	193
New vaccines	197
Natural selection and vaccines	198
Animal vaccines	194
References	205
Epilogue	219

New vaccines are being invented every year, all with the same hope - to be included in the Immunization Schedule. It's very big money. There is no reason to believe we'll stop now at 68 vaccines mandated before a child is eighteen. But infant mortality rates and the health of our children are appalling. The incidence of both infectious diseases and degenerative diseases among Americans is skyrocketing.

Declining health among school children is obvious. Ritalin, insulin, antidepressants, and inhalers are rampant in our schools. Despite the highest intake of antibiotics and vaccines of any group of children in history, our kids are fatter, sicker, and dumber than ever before. (Harvard School [76] [34])

Child obesity is 37%; with 60% overweight. Quoting CDC figures for asthma incidence, since 1980 asthma more than doubled and is right on track to double again by 2020. [178, 73]

Most of the increase is in children, who account for more than 12 million cases. (Borenstein) [187]) More than 8.9% of US children have **asthma**. [111, *National Center*] In some schools, one out of four kids is walking around with an inhaler. The news usually focuses on what a big mystery asthma is even though we're spending some **$20 billion** per year to treat it. [112, ALA]

The number of abnormal children is shocking: 13% of American public school children are enrolled in programs for some type of disability. [91] More than **15 million** US children are learning disabled. [92]

At least **one in six** American children has a neurodevelopmental disorder! (Geier - IOM hearings [105])

SAT indices have been "re-centered" twice in the past 8 years in order to make it look as though high school kids aren't as ignorant as they really are. [34] Exit exams are made easier and easier, following the delusional 'no child left behind' policy.

OPTING OUT

A growing number of medical researchers and doctors disagree with the 68 vaccinations that children are required to get. [303] More parents are opting out by signing exemption forms. They're drawing the line. They're saying, if nothing else is sacred in this world, at least the blood of our children should not be subject to the whims of politics and big money. That bloodstream should only be violated in life-threatening situations. And never with anything experimental or unproven or dangerous.

Most of what is written about the subject insists that vaccines are safe, effective, and necessary. We hear how modern civilization has been saved from the ravages of infectious disease by the intervention of miraculous vaccines. We hear how important it is for children to get their shots so they'll be safe from disease, etc. We keep hearing about new vaccines that are supposedly necessary to defend against new diseases.

How can both viewpoints be right? These are two conflicting views on the nature of biological reality. Both sides often get very shrill, emotional, and unscientific; such a chasm widens between them that is profoundly disconcerting. But someone is wrong:

Either

vaccines are essential for our children's health and safety

or

vaccines are weakening and poisoning our children.

There is so much false reporting and badly referenced data on both sides of the debate that the concerned parent must eventually ask: What do we really know for sure about any of this?

A MODEST PROPOSAL

It's no metaphor to say that the bloodstream of our children is the future of our civilization. Such an environment should be guarded. This chapter proposes the following condition - before we put anything into that bloodstream, we should be quite sure

1. **the child's health demands it**
2. **no chance of harm**

Such common sense as this comes off as radical to the undiscriminating American public, who in general seem to have lost the ability for rational discourse and taking responsibility for their own children's well being.

A NEW EVENT IN HUMAN HISTORY

arrived with the advent of vaccines: mandatory administration, enforced by legislation. Government began claiming a right over the bloodstream of its citizens. Unless parents sign exemption forms, children must be vaccinated before they get into school. Legislation is controlled by lobbying. And the most powerful lobby in Washington is the pharmaceutical industry. [102]

Now that's vexing already - what's the prime criterion going to be: corporate profits or proven health benefits for our children? If a choice has to be made, which one will defer to the other?

NOT MY JOB

Many parents starting to read this will say - Oh I don't need to know any of that stuff. That's my doctor's job to know it. Two problems with that:

    1. Many doctors don't know it.

    2. Many doctors who do know don't vaccinate their own children. But they will vaccinate yours.   [303]

In this chapter you will be getting primarily the minority view, but one which has abundant support and documentation, and which anyone taking children in for shots needs to know about. When you get to something you totally doubt, please do two things:

    1. check the references
    2. follow the money

MILKING THE SACRED COW

Vaccination is a very powerful and emotionally charged issue, with enormous political considerations. To make a responsible decision in the best interests of the child, one must be willing to question a paradigm learned over a lifetime of conditioning.

But for some reason, resistance to correct information about vaccination often resembles religious fanaticism. Unlike with

Ritalin, Lipitor, or antibiotics, people seem to get violently emotional about vaccinations, with a blind, hysterical zeal. There are many cases today where social services actually take children away from parents who were exercising their legal right to exempt the child from vaccination.

Why the histrionics? Why are vaccines such a Sacred Cow? Why do they expend so much effort

KEEPING THE LID ON?

As in any area served by billion dollar industries, information on vaccination is very controlled. Setting out to try and discover the truth about vaccines, one is not prepared for the extent of systematic misdirection, nor for the amount of documentation opposing vaccination, much of it from top medical sources. After awhile, it's hard to decide whom to believe: either the body can learn its own immunity, or else it is enormously inadequate, and requires help from the genius of medical science for survival.

MEDSPEAK

Our programming starts with two simple words: vaccination and immunization. We're trained to think of them as synonyms, right? That's no accident. What's the difference?

Immunization means the body becomes immune to something, all by itself. That only happens after getting a disease, or at least being exposed to it. **Vaccination**, by contrast, just means to stick a needle into someone's arm and inject a manmade substance we call vaccine. Entirely different ballgame. Now that you know the difference, stop saying immunization when you mean vaccination.

The use of the word 'immunization' instead of 'vaccination' is pervasive within both medical and popular literature, pretending a semantic equivalence between the two terms. Predictably, it has now become rare to find references to 'vaccination' in medical literature, even though that is the correct term. Big difference here. Start noticing.

WHAT IS A VACCINE?

> "a suspension of attenuated or killed microorganisms
> ...administered for prevention ...or treatment of disease."
> - Dorland's *Medical Dictionary* p 696 [208]

From a cow - that was the original root of the word itself. We will see if vaccines can prevent or treat anything.

MONEY AND VACCINES

What kind of money are we talking about with vaccines?

Back in 1993, worldwide vaccines were

> "...about a **$3 billion** a year industry... dominated by large
> multinational corporations, such as Merck, Pasteur-Merieux-
> Connaught, Biocine-Sclavo, Smith-KlineBeecham and Wyeth."
> - Philip K. Russell, MD   [205]

Two years later, **$4 billion**. [97] By 2003, **$6 billion**. By 2005 world sales topped **$8 billion** annually. [120]

The cost of vaccine purchase in the year 2020 following the

recommendation of 7 additional vaccines was estimated to be $1225 per child. (*Am Journal of Pub Health* 2002) [164]   But we're way past that. We've added 28 childhood vaccines since 2002.

By Feb 2004 we were up to $606 per child.   ([107]] CDC)

Here's a summary of money spent **per child** on vaccines:

1975	**$10**
2001	**$385**
2004	**$606**
2011	**$1200+**

TOTAL GLOBAL VACCINE SPENDING: BEST GUESS

Today it has become very difficult to pinpoint total global vaccine expenditures. Recent government figures estimate **$23 billion** by 2012 [67] (*GAO Report to Congress*) which number has been parroted by various sources since 2007. Or there's the *Forbes* magazine Lehman Brothers figure of **$30 billion**. [322].

The lowball inaccuracy of such guesses stems from their exclusion of global R&D money, Third World experimentation, vaccines as foreign aid programs, vaccines in the developmental pipeline, etc., in looking at the whole picture. Citing only the sales figures of actual vaccines does not accurately reflect the magnitude of the entire global vaccine industry, of which a reasonable estimate today is certainly in excess of **$50 billion** per annum, all in.

In Feb 2010 Bill Gates ante-ed up his $10 billion in vaccines for one reason: return on investment. [36]   Coupled with his bizarre admission that vaccines are one of the 3 best ways to reduce world population, his success is all but assured. (video, [37])

THE REAL GREEN

From the World Health Organization's 2006 figures we discover that just in developing countries there were

43 million injections given per day
16 billion injections per year   [90]

A lot more than vaccines is at stake here.   Vaccines are the foundation of the entire Well Baby program - the livelihood of the whole pediatric industry. That's many billion$. If a child doesn't go in for his shots, look at all those missed opportunities to upsell the parents on eartubes, antibiotics, and a host of other drugs and procedures. Consider how growing up without vaccines is a huge economic threat. The Well Baby Program introduces a human being to a lifetime of dependency on organized medicine. If a child can grow up healthy without doctors and drugs, this posits the dangerous concepts of self-reliance and trust in the body's own natural healing powers.

RESERVOIRS FOR DISEASE

Be advised: this Orwellian buzzphrase is the product of some very sophisticated drug industry think-tank ruminations. Reservoirs for disease: the fantasy being that the unvaccinated are unprotected from disease and are therefore a collective breeding ground that threatens the vaccinated. Throughout this book the exact opposite will be proven again and again: it is the vaccinated children in this country whose immune systems are being systematically suppressed, whose inner milieu is a viable medium for opportunistic organisms, even though they are now receiving more vaccines than any group of children in the history of the world.

HISTORY -- PART I

SMALLPOX - THE BIRTH OF VACCINE

Smallpox was an infectious viral disease evident for centuries in places with poor sanitation, poverty, and malnutrition. Hundreds of thousands died, and there was no cure. The infectious agent was called *Orthopox variola*. [160] By the end of the 18th century the disease was following the usual natural course: burning itself out on the human population, confining itself to those with the lowest immune capabilities, and mutating. Herd immunity.

Smallpox was commonly regarded as divine punishment for unnamed errors. It never occurred to people that overcrowding, poor hygiene, contaminated food and water, or poor nutrition had anything to do with it. A superstition then emerged that milkmaids who contracted a mild disease known as cowpox were thereby immune to smallpox.

EDWARD JENNER

as you may remember, was the English "physician" in the late 1700s who made use of that old superstition. As an experiment, Jenner came up with the idea of drawing serum from a cowpox pustule on the skin of an infected milkmaid – 9 year old Sarah

Nelmes. [295, Miller] He was then reckless enough to actually inoculate the infected pus into another subject, on the theory that contact with this "milder" disease would allow the subject to develop immunity to the more deadly smallpox.

Jenner's wild theory was that this cow-pox is smallpox of the cow. Therefore, if you give a person cowpox, it is the same as smallpox, only in a very mild form. And it would not be infectious.

Going even farther out on a limb, Jenner himself then declared that it is not that cowpox is preventive of smallpox but that it **is** smallpox itself! (*Enquiry*, 1798 [162])

After inoculating his very first patient - 8 year old James Phipps - Jenner absurdly maintained that his injections were conferring lifetime immunity:

   "...what renders the cowpox virus so extremely singular is that the person who has been thus affected is forever after secure from the infection of the smallpox."
                           - Jenner, 1797, cited in H.B. Anderson [204]

NOT SO FAST

While Jenner is universally venerated today as mankind's deliverer from the scourge of smallpox in probably 99% of sources because of his "discovery" of inoculation, what most edited modern drafts of the story omit is the

   - utter lack of science behind Jenner's original claim of
       immunity from vaccines

- recklessness in producing smallpox vaccine
- number of deaths and disfiguring cases from his injections

REALITY CHECK

Many of Jenner's own contemporaries were shocked at how easily the scientific community was taken in by this poser. Perusing the work of Walter Hadwen MD, celebrated English surgeon, author, and medical scholar of 100 years ago, we find a version of the Jenner story that is not quite so cast in bronze as what we have always been told. Hadwen points out a few cracks in Jenner's pedestal: [191]

- Jenner was no physician. He never completed any program of medical study, or received a diploma from any medical school. If you go to the Jenner Museum in Gloucestershire, England today and ask for Jenner's diploma, you will be told "we don't have it."

- Jenner bought his medical degree for £15 from St Andrew's College in Scotland, which he never attended. (Hume, p 174 [202], also Hadwen [191, 192])

- Jenner "tested" his theory on one patient, and immediately claimed that he had "immunized" the patient against smallpox for life. Jenner then claimed that it would work universally. That's it! No controlled clinical trials, no years of research, nothing.

Modern whitewashed versions of the story never mention that James Phipps died at age 20, having been inoculated with vaccine each year! Or that Jenner's own son died at 21, also revaccinated over and over. (Baron, vol 2 [225])

With no proof whatsoever, Jenner tricked the entire medical profession, then and now, into pretending that cowpox was smallpox in cows - a total scientific inaccuracy. And then he sold the idea that his vaccine was the cure. [192, 272]

WHEEL OF FORTUNE

A few years after his "breakthrough," Jenner's repeated petitions to the House of Commons struck gold, or actually sterling. It finally dawned on the English government how millions of pounds could change hands by passing a law making Jenner's smallpox vaccine compulsory. Jenner was promptly awarded the enormous sum of £30,000 by British Parliament and suddenly this uncredentialed primadonna was a revered scientist. [193]

Soon Parliament began passing laws to make the untested vaccine compulsory throughout the British empire. The rest of Europe soon followed suit.

Once the economic implications of compulsory vaccinations were realized, dissenting voices went unpublished. Then as now, the media were largely controlled by vaccine manufacturers and the government, who stood to make huge money from the sale of these absurd vaccines. Hadwen put it like this: [272]

"... so strong is the effect of authority, custom, and endowment, and so prone are people to save themselves the trouble of personal investigation by the simple process of accepting the decisions of "the majority" ...

"When once an error is accepted by a profession and endowed by Government, to uproot it becomes a herculean task."

Sound familiar? Despite the lack of scientific validation and the tens of thousands of documented vaccine deaths, compulsory smallpox vaccination lasted for 120 years!   And then in 2002 America geared up to do it all again.

TWO DIFFERENT DISEASES

Let's back up a moment and look at the original science. In the first place, these two diseases - **cowpox** and **smallpox** - are two completely distinct conditions, as Hadwen explains:

"What is **cow-pox**? It is a disease which occurs on the teats of cows; it only occurs when they are in milk; only in one part of the body, and naturally only in the female animal; it results in an ugly chancre; and is not infectious.

"**Small-pox**, on the other hand, is not limited to the female sex as is cow-pox, nor to one portion of the body; it presents different physical signs, and, furthermore, is tremendously infectious, and the course and symptoms of the two diseases are totally different.

"Therefore there is no analogy between the two." [192]

Legitimate scientists of Jenner's day, like Bechamp, Hadwen, Wallace, and others thought it appalling that these distinctions between cowpox and smallpox were never discussed. If the axioms of immunology were true, how could one disease bug immunize against a completely separate disease?

Doing a taxonomic check in a standard index of viruses from a National Institutes of Health database [273] readily points out that cowpox is linked with a virus called *Orthopox vaccinia* and smallpox with a virus called *Orthopox variola*. These two viruses have different sizes, genetic sequences, and characteristics.

They're different species. To pretend that cows get a version of smallpox called cowpox is bizarre enough - but then to say that people who get the same disease are thereby immune to smallpox is utterly fictional.

This chart may be helpful: (*Microsoft Encarta* [175])

Cowpox	**Smallpox**
In cows	**In humans**
Not infectious to cows	**Infectious to humans**
Orthopox vaccinia	*Orthopox variola*

Here's how modern science glosses over the apparent contradiction, perpetuating the fable: From *The Columbia Encyclopedia*, Sixth Edition: [176] **cowpox**:

"... infectious disease of cows caused by a virus related to the virus of smallpox. Also called **variola**, it is characterized by pustular lesions on the teats and udder. Cowpox is transmitted by contact, inducing a mild infection of the hands in persons who milk infected cows. The fact that such persons had immunity to smallpox led Edward Jenner to attempt vaccination with this virus, instead of using the dangerous method of vaccinating with material from the sores of smallpox. Jenner's method was successful and is the basis of the modern vaccination against smallpox."

The majority of historical references have loudly proclaimed the sound science behind smallpox vaccine, up to the present day.

SMALLPOX OR COWPOX?

From an *MSN Encarta* document:

"**Cowpox**, contagious viral disease of cows characterized by pustular eruptions. Cowpox can be transmitted to humans by direct contact. Persons infected with cowpox become immune to smallpox, a similar but more serious disease. This immunity was discovered by Edward Jenner, who used cowpox virus to inoculate patients against smallpox."   - "Cowpox,"   [175]

ONLY IN HORSESHOES AND HAND GRENADES

Why have all smallpox vaccines since the time of Jenner contained the wrong virus? Entrenched medical error. The 2002 smallpox vaccines - Dryvax and Acambis' ACAM1000 - still contained *Orthopox vaccinia*, not *Orthopox variola*. (*NEJM*, [156], [165], King [136]) Smallpox is the only vaccine for which this 'close cousin' ruse has ever been tried.

As we saw in *The Doors of Perception* [301], the molders of the public mind are banking that most people will never look below the surface to discover the unscientific and illogical basis for issues which have huge economic significance. Everybody knows that in America people just don't read any more.

FORGOTTEN CONCOCTIONS OF SMALLPOX VACCINE

On the way to becoming the dangerous and useless product it is today, smallpox vaccine has been true to its origins. Here are a few of the other sources from which Jenner and others drew the material which they also claimed was smallpox vaccine, up until 1898:

> - infected horse hooves
> - pustules on cows who had been infected with human
>   smallpox
> - pustules on humans who had been deliberately
>   infected with horse grease and cowpox
> - pustules on humans infected with smallpox
>   - (Baxby [224], *An Enquiry* [163], [295])

Horse grease was the name of a hoof infection disease. Jenner felt justified in injecting pus from infected horse hooves into healthy children because he dreamed up the notion that cowpox was harbored in the infected hooves. [163]   Not kidding.

Guess where Jenner got smallpox pus for his vaccine. Give up? Human corpses, dead from smallpox! [276]

For over 150 years, there was virtually no consistency in the preparation of smallpox vaccine. [296]

Turns out that cowpox itself is not a natural disease of cows. Cowpox is a disease of the udder which came about by farmers milking the cows with filthy hands. Often after having just cleaned infections in other animals, or after any other farm chore for that matter. Syphilis and tuberculosis were commonly present in the pustular cowpox lesions from which the precious "vaccine" was extracted. ([195], SAV [296], [295])

Another popular Jennerian method was the **arm-to-arm** technique. (Rains [194]) Until it became illegal in 1898, pustular material was simply drawn from a corpse's arm and inoculated into a patient. The reason for the 1898 law was to curb the rampant transmission of syphilis and tuberculosis. (Baxby [224])

In reading these old histories, one gradually realizes that many of the "vaccines" didn't go through any manufacturing steps or preparation whatsoever. Before 1856, a large percentage of the early smallpox vaccines were nothing more than arbitrary jabs of human and animal pus directly into a healthy child's bloodstream! (SAV [296], whale.to [292])

THE BLOOD OF ANIMALS

Here we see the level of the science underlying smallpox vaccine for the past two centuries. The random cross-mixing of blood between man and animals violated common traditions and taboos of most cultures from time immemorial. Most religions specifically forbade it. Cowpox was not a natural disease in cows; syphilis was not a natural disease in man. Smallpox was not a natural disease in cows, nor in any other animals: it had to be injected into them. How many other diseases have their roots in this quixotic inter-species experimentation? Bad ju-ju to ignore Mother Nature.

By 1875, smallpox vaccine had become so crossed and intermixed from so many different sources, passed through so many different species, that the actual composition was truly unknown. There was no consistency worldwide - in any location smallpox vaccine was whatever the local authorities said it was. Any given smallpox vaccine might have its origins in goat pox, swine pox, cowpox, monkeypox, horse grease, human smallpox or any combination thereof. [296]

DID THE VACCINE WORK? PRUSSIAN ROULETTE

By 1853, Parliament began passing laws to make the untested vaccine compulsory throughout the British empire. Other countries of Europe followed suit.

Dr Hadwen provides a rare window into the medical research of a century ago, one that has not received the usual whitewash. He tells the amazing story about Prussia, the most vaccinated country in Europe during the 1800s, and the country which kept the best records. Hadwen had access to these medical records before the media had the sense to suppress them. Here's what they showed: ([272, 276])

It happened that Prussia passed a mandatory vaccination law in **1834** for smallpox. The law provided that every infant be vaccinated, and then revaccinated when starting school. After graduation he had to be vaccinated again, and then once more upon entering the Army. And all healthy males had to go into the Army. Anyone who refused the vaccination was to be "held down and vaccinated by force; and so thoroughly was it done that he was then vaccinated in **ten places** on each arm." [272]

OK, so we get the idea that almost 100% of Prussians got Jenner's smallpox vaccine. So what happened in Prussia 35 years after this vaccination law? A smallpox epidemic of **1 million cases** which killed "**124,978** of her vaccinated and re-vaccinated citizens after thirty-five years of compulsory vaccination!"

LICENCE TO KILL

How about England?

A compulsory "immunization" program was set up in England in **1853** using Jenner's methods. (McBean p.13)[211] Before that time, the highest number of deaths in a 2 year period in England from smallpox was about **2000**.

Results of this "immunization":

year	deaths
1857-9	14,244
1863-5	20,059

In response, in 1867 Parliament enacted a stricter vaccination law, and **97%** of the people were inoculated. New result:

year	deaths	
1868	44,840	- Null, Part III, p 23 [220]

Excellent vaccine, what?

Alfred Russell Wallace offers abundant proof how vaccine statistics were manipulated in England during the 1800s - the who and the why of it. After thoroughly charting actual deaths throughout the UK and the Continent from smallpox and from the vaccine, Wallace concludes that smallpox vaccine

"...has actually **increased susceptibility** to the disease. ... the conclusion is in every case the same: that vaccination is a gigantic

delusion; that it has never saved a single life; but that it has been the cause of so much disease, so many deaths, such a vast amount of utterly needless and altogether undeserved suffering, that it will be classed by the coming generation among the greatest errors of an ignorant and prejudiced age, the foulest blot on ... our century."
                    - Alfred R. Wallace, Chapter VI 1898   [193]

PHILIPPINE FIASCO

After WWI, there was a lot of surplus smallpox vaccine that didn't get used. So we looked to another market we could control. When the U.S. mandated a mass smallpox vaccination program in the Philippines in 1917, some **25 million shots** were given to those people. **163,000** Filipinos came down with the disease after the vaccination, and **75,339** of them died from it, **quadrupling** the death rate prior to the inoculation program. That's far more than the total number of Americans who died in the entire Vietnam war! American "immunization" of its Philippine territory caused several horrific epidemics there that didn't quite make the six o'clock news. (Anderson, p 69 W.H.Hay, also James, p 410 [204, 221, 199])

SLOW LEARNERS

What most people don't know is that just after the US began vaccinating for smallpox (1902) England stopped. By 1907 England had no more compulsory smallpox vaccination. Holland, same thing in 1928. Australia – 1925. ([204], p 10)

How long did it take the US to figure it out? We finally stopped in 1971, the last holdout in the world.

The low ebb of the infectious diseases arrived in the 1970s. From

1950 to 1970, **zero** cases of smallpox were reported in the U.S. After 1970, there were a few cases of smallpox, but they only occurred among the ranks of the vaccinated! (Scheibner) [239]

What's important to notice is that smallpox vaccination in the U.S. persisted another **30 years** after the disease was at an incidence of practically zero. Again, **the only source of death from smallpox in the U.S. for 30 years was from the vaccine itself**. (Mendelsohn, p 232; *World Book*, 1994) [241, 245]

Today smallpox occurs nowhere in nature.

FAIRY TALES CAN COME TRUE

To sum up, what Jenner really did was to take an old superstition of Gloucester dairymaids and pander it into an enormous fortune for himself and the English government by the most unfounded "scientific" posturing. [177]

SMALLPOX POST 9/11

From 9/11 until early 2003, popular media employed a brilliant menage of pseudoscience and well-edited history to concoct a new myth out of thin air: terrorists were about to release smallpox as a bioweapon that could decimate our population. Government leaders with degrees in law, not science, decided to prepare enough vaccine to inoculate every American. And to empower themselves to legislate the vaccine's administration, sanctioned by severe penalties for refusal. (Altman [131])

Price tag for the new doses: over **$3 billion**. But what is money when compared with the health and security of the American people?

Answer: it's still money.

Post-9/11 politics created marketing niches the likes of which the world had never seen.

The illusion of a smallpox threat was crafted - a $3 billion dream. [125] Throughout 2002, the unlettered public were unrelentingly terrorized with media scenarios of crazed Muslims unleashing weaponized smallpox into metropolitan areas, supposedly resulting in epidemics of smallpox spreading like wildfire through an unvaccinated population, etc. Remember?

Despite all this, the FDA, CDC, HHS, Office of Homeland Security, plus many of the new offices which suddenly emerged at the trough, decided that a few companies should produce enough vaccine to give all 280 million Americans 'protection.' [297] The companies included Aventis in France, Acambis in England, and Wyeth in the US.

THE HOUSE OF CARDS BEGINS TO QUAKE

On 10 Sept 02 with the CDC announced that the new smallpox vaccine was not to be recommended for:

   - HIV people
   - anyone on immunosuppressive drugs
   - anyone with eczema   [158]

The CDC quoted a study in the *Journal of Allergy and Clinical Immunology*, describing vaccine reactions like blindness, scarring, and death. How many Americans would be excluded?

"Given the number of people who suffer from eczema, up to **one half** of the US population may be ineligible for routine smallpox vaccination." **[152]**

AIDS patients and those on immunosuppressive drugs add another significant proportion to the group of those who shouldn't be vaccinated.   Let's see - how many drugs are immuno-suppressive?   Like, all of them?

Most Americans over 31 years of age had already been vaccinated for smallpox, since the vaccine was only halted in 1971 in the US. So if the vaccine really worked, then obviously these people will not need a new shot, right?

SMALLPOX HEART ATTACKS

The final nail in the coffin for the post 9/11 smallpox vaccine program was the discovery in Mar 2003 that the vaccine should not be given to heart patients.   [138] [139]

The same individual who invented the program finally pulled it:

"Under the new guidelines, people who have been diagnosed with serious heart disease such as coronary artery disease, congestive heart failure, heart attack and angina are being told not to get the vaccine. The change was ordered by Health and Human Services Secretary Tommy Thompson."   [138]

All this wasn't discovered until after the $3 billion was spent.

So whom did that leave eligible for the vaccine?   **Ten per cent** of the population would be a reasonable estimate.

THE CASE OF THE DISAPPEARING THREAT

The program of mass smallpox vaccination was officially abandoned in Oct 2003. According to Ray Strikas of the CDC:

"the much-ballyhooed program is dead in the water." [119]

Reason: heart complications, and the above problems. So after 2 years of terrorizing the public with the threat of forced inoculations and after spending $3 billion, they axe the whole thing, just like that. So what about the bioterrorist threat of smallpox? Where did it go? Why didn't they talk about it any more? Does that mean it only had reality as a marketing tool for the vaccine, but since the vaccine's no good, then the threat disappears too? What a polite pathogen, to back off just because we couldn't find a cure.

HISTORY -- PART II

PASTEUR - THE LUCKY CHEMIST

After Jenner, the next big name in vaccines was Pasteur. Louis Pasteur was a French chemist in the mid 1800s, one of a group of scientists in both France and Germany who were grappling with fundamental questions about life:

- what makes something alive?
- where do germs come from?
- which comes first, germ or disease?
- why do things rot, ferment, or decompose?

For the first time in history, discoveries were being made about these elementary issues. Ideas were coming fast, but piecemeal. It was perfect timing for an opportunist to take advantage of the general uncertainty and to claim that he understood all the issues involved, and furthermore had thought of them first. Pasteur was known for his habit of playing both sides of the fence on issues he didn't understand, and then later, to quote only the parts of his early writings that supported the later finding, always with the claim that he had been there first. Only scientists studied the complexities of these emerging ideas. The royal court and the press just knew that something was going on, and though they didn't know what, were going to act as though they did. Same as now. For them, a chameleon like Pasteur was the perfect frontman.

Once it became clear which way the winds of fortune were blowing. Pasteur saw his way to a career behind a new dogma:

THE GERM THEORY OF DISEASE

What exactly was this Germ Theory? Very simply, the Germ Theory holds that there are separate diseases and that each disease is caused by a particular microorganism. It was the job of science, then, to find the right drug or vaccine that will selectively kill off the offending bug without killing the patient.

That would be great, but rarely is nature so black and white about things, ever notice that? For one thing, bacteria and viruses tend to be picky about their environments. That's why some people get colds and others don't. That's why some survived the Bubonic Plague. That's also why some doctors and nurses seem to be immune to disease even though they're surrounded by it every day.

Deepak Chopra tells us of a study in which the influenza virus was isolated and implanted directly onto the mucous membranes of a group of subjects, with only 12% of them getting the flu. (*Quantum Healing* [262])

Disease happens when systems of the body become so weak and nutrient-starved that they shut down. What causes that? Low resistance, filth, toxic diet, bad lifestyle, weak immune system. Such imbalance renders the blood a hospitable medium in which opportunist organisms may be cultured. Eventually even Pasteur agreed that bugs - bacteria and viruses - do not cause disease, but rather are the scavengers of diseased tissue.

The Germ Theory has as many holes as a Swiss cheese, and Pasteur knew it. But a little research shows us that Pasteur had a rare gift for PR. He never missed the occasion to court magistrates, noblemen, and legislators in the drawing rooms of Europe. Dealing with scientific matters incompletely understood even by Pasteur himself, the members of the aristocracy tended to accept Pasteur's version of current science. [202]

When the Brass Ring of mass vaccination eventually occurred to the government leaders, Pasteur was primed.

PASTEUR UNMASKED

There was a unique book published in 1923 that is still in print: *Bechamp or Pasteur?* This book was written by E. Douglas Hume, who it turns out was actually a woman who had to disguise her name to get the book published.

Hume serves up a few beguiling morsels about Pasteur:

- Pasteur had no training or credentials in either medicine or physiology; he was a chemist

- Pasteur very likely created the disease known as hydrophobia, (rabies) rather than found a cure for it.

- Pasteur initiated the practice of **vivisection** with horrific animal experiments. Hundreds of thousands of laboratory animals have been needlessly killed by atrocious experiments in the name of "science," throughout the entire empire of medical research laboratories worldwide, even to the present time.

- Rather than protecting the human race from disease, Pasteur may be seen more as a merchant than a scientist, with his frequent reporting of false test findings.

GERMS: THE EVIDENCE OF DISEASE, NOT THE CAUSE

As far as Pasteur's Germ Theory goes, there was much opposition to it among leading scientists of his own time.

Perhaps the greatest scientist in France during Pasteur's time, the discoverer of bacteria was Antoine Bechamp, University of Lille. Dr Bechamp said: [211], p183

"Bacteria do not cause disease, and therefore serums and vaccines can neither prevent nor cure disease."

The author of the cell theory, Rudolf Virchow himself, agreed:

"Germs seek their natural habitat – diseased tissue – rather than being the cause of diseased tissue."
                                                   - Man the Unknown [278]

SCAVENGERS NOT PREDATORS

Along with many other scientists then and now, Virchow realized that the presence of germs may identify the tissue as diseased, but did not necessarily **create** the diseased condition. Weakened or diseased tissue is a target area for microorganisms, a hospitable environment in which opportunists can set up shop. But that's quite different from predatory germs having caused the weakened state. First the patient gets sick; germs show up later.

Authors and doctors enslaved to the Germ Theory today are still playing their only trump card – Alexander Fleming's discovery of penicillin in 1928. They are desperately hoping for a reprise of medicine's greatest triumph. No one would be more embarrassed by their invocations than Fleming himself, who predicted the rise of the superbugs by reckless overprescription of antibiotics - our wildly unscientific 'just in case' policy. [99]

A DRUG FOR EVERY BUG

The militaristic idea that the normal human condition is to live in this hermetically-sealed antiseptic little capsule in which all other life forms must be regarded as invaders and killed off – this notion is scientifically untenable, even though it is the lodestone of modern medicine.

Healthy humans subsist in a biosphere, surrounded by thousands of microbes, both internally and externally, all co-existing in a dynamic equilibrium that is beneficial to all participants.

Dr Khem Shahani, premier authority on intestinal probiotics, proved that the normal human colon should contain up to 3 lbs of flora – as many as 400 different species. [101] There are species of microscopic spiders who live their entire lifespan on the human eyelash. [313]   Dr Alec Burton proved that tetanus bacillus is found on the skin and even in the mouths of ordinary healthy individuals without causing disease. [305]

Legitimate scientists see germ proliferation not as the cause of disease but rather the evidence of disease. The disease came first. This simple concept, which organized medicine /your pediatrician cannot discuss, is really the key idea of this book.

ON WITH THE SHOW

Politics never changes. The same type of thinking that kept Galileo under house arrest for discovering that the earth went around the sun, the rulers' eternal attempt to control the minds of their subjects, these are the forces that cast Pasteur, an ambitious opportunist, into a role he may not have deserved - the imagined Trailblazer in the science of modern biomedicine.

Howard Hencke, in his 1995 book *The Germ Theory: A Deliberate Aberration,* notes that the Germ Theory wanted   [279]

"... to indoctrinate the public in the Western world with the belief that the salvation from all, especially physical ailments, lay outside the individual's system and responsibility, because it was caused by external factors... and that chemical remedies will keep him free from disease, independent of his own vigilant responsibility."

We're talking marketing here, yes?

"Had it not been for the mass selling of vaccines, Pasteur's germ theory of disease would have collapsed into obscurity."

- E. Douglas Hume   [202]

INVIOLABLE ENVIRONMENT

From the beginning, the whole idea of piercing the skin with a needle for any reason was suspect, let alone introducing new proteins and agents into what was supposed to be an inviolable environment: the circulatory system. We just assume injecting microbes into the infant's blood is safe and scientific, without giving it a second thought. Popular media and scientific literature always make this unfounded assumption. But injections are a total **violation** of nature. It was nature's design that nothing be introduced into the bloodstream without going through the laboratory of the digestive or respiratory systems. It's never scientific to defile nature, no matter how they may spin it.

Isn't this common sense? Ever think about the instincts of infants and children when they see a syringe? Why wouldn't we trust those instincts? You want to use the it's-for-their-own-good slogan, well then, you better know what you're talking about.

Among the dozens of scientists opposing inoculation:

"The most serious disorders may be provoked by the injection of living organisms into the blood... into a medium not intended

for them may provoke redoubtable manifestations of the gravest morbid phenomena."

- Antoine Bechamp [202]

Reporting from the battlefields of South Africa during the Boer War in the early part of last century, Walter Hadwen, MD, in his book *Microbes and War* notes that the war itself killed 86,000 men. With a 100% inoculation rate, there were an **additional** 96,000 casualties from disease alone! [280]

ILLOGICAL RATIONALE

Pasteur began the practice of vivisection with horrific animal experiments, which have never been proven valid. Would you give your cat your cold medicine? In the natural state, animals have different diseases from humans, and rarely. This one error has led us down a costly and ultimately fruitless path. How can we hope to cure human disease by giving animals diseases they would never have gotten in nature, then pretending that such diseases are the same ones we get, and then seeing which drugs cover up the animal's symptoms? Then we smugly conclude that those same drugs will have the same effect in humans! Idiotic as that sounds, it's precisely what we do. Animal testing remains the basis for the entire empire of medical research, publication, and the whole approval process for prescription drugs. (Hans Ruesch) [281]

WHOLE NEW MARKET

One concept we should not gloss over, of pivotal importance in understanding how and why vaccines came about: **For the first time in history, doctors would no longer confine themselves to**

the sick. With vaccines, doctors are now going to claim that perfectly healthy people need the injections in order to stay healthy.

Selling such an impossibly fanciful concept obviously would require wagging some major dog. As masters of the scientific universe, doctors will pretend they are fortunate enough to have unlocked the hidden health secrets of the ages, which they now will mercifully share with a grateful humanity. For a price.

WHAT'S IN VACCINES?

Although the complete composition of today's vaccines are secret formulae, protected by law as proprietary intel, many of the ingredients are listed in the *Physicians Desk Reference*, in each vaccine's section. This is their version of disclosure.

From this limited viewpoint, we can see some of the main ingredients:

attenuated pathogens
toxoids
adjuvants
preservatives
excipients

The full strength microbe is not used in vaccines, but rather a weakened, half-killed mutation - the **attenuated** version.

A **toxoid** is a poisonous excretion of a pathogen which is claimed to be able to trigger immunity, since it came from the original bug.

An **adjuvant** is a poisonous compound like formaldehyde, ethylene glycol, or mercury which is used to provoke a stronger immune response than would be evoked from the attenuated pathogen alone.   (Burnet p. 85) [201]

This problem with this notion is that provoking an immune response is totally different from conferring some beneficial lasting immunity. This is a fundamental flaw in the whole vaccine argument, which nobody talks about.

The first vaccines by Jenner and Pasteur, and also most modern ones, are experimental proteins made from rotting, diseased samples of animal tissue (**cows, birds, sheep, monkeys, guinea pigs, humans, and horses**) carrying some weakened infectious agent.

Components like **formaldehyde, aluminum, mercury, ethylene glycol,** which are euphemistically called **adjuvants,** or helpers, in reality help nothing but the toxicity of the vaccine. That is, how much of an immune kick it sparks. (*PDR* 2010)[75] But the strength of immune response has no proven effect on enhancing health or immunity.

Mercury is in the form of thimerosal. Minute traces of mercury can cause permanent nerve damage and autoimmune disorders.

Formaldehyde is a carcinogenic embalming fluid. (*PDR* p1383 [244]) Aluminum is a potent neurotoxin, which can cause much more neurologic mischief than just Alzheimer's disease. [180, 249]

Excipients are oil compounds used as carriers to prolong and enhance the immune effect. Unfortunately the refined oils still contain intact proteins, which in children cause epidemic food sensitivity and even anaphylaxis. [16]

The companies are not required to disclose all the ingredients, protected by issues of intellectual property. Vaccines today are some of the most closely guarded of all industrial secrets. The cold reality is that parents really have no way of knowing exactly what is being injected into their children.

That's a lot of trust to ask, especially after looking at the track record of the companies, as we do throughout this book. Not to mention their exemption from liability.

CULTURE MEDIA

The active part of a vaccine is a disease organism which is grown or cultured on a certain medium. Here are some of the culture media for today's vaccines, as listed in the 2011 *PDR*:   [9]

lung cells of aborted human fetus   human blood
kidneys of African green monkeys   diphtheria cultures
infected human connective tissue   infected animal cells
(monkey, pig, calf, canary, rabbit, chicken, guinea pig)

Why are we not horrified by the above list? Why such a shrill insistence that vaccinations are safe, in the absence of scientific evidence? Maybe it's our primordial, tribal fascination with superstitions involving parts and extracts and entrails from dead animals. These beliefs harken forth from the dawn of humanity, and are cited in the chronicles of most civilizations. They're imprinted on the hard disk of our primitive brain.

Medical thinking is that if the patient gets a minor case of the disease under the "controlled" conditions of vaccination, he will produce his own **antibodies** to the vaccine, which will confer lifetime immunity by remembering what the bad bug looks like the next time it shows up, and then neutralizing it. [320]

But there's a little more to it than that.

SIMPLISTIC PARADIGM: ANTIGEN/ANTIBODY

First off, there is no general agreement that the vaccine-antibody paradigm is really the whole story of immunity. Researchers like Alan Phillips, founding director of Citizens for Health Care and Freedom, realize that   [240]

"natural immunity is a complex phenomenon involving many organs and systems; it cannot be fully replicated by the artificial stimulation of antibody production."

Dr. Gerald Edelman won the Nobel prize for his discovery that the immune system doesn't operate solely on the popular antigen-antibody model. Edelman showed that hundreds of antibodies are already present at birth, having evolved within our species over the centuries. ([159] p 17)

Natural immunity is a much more complex subject than the vaccine salesmen would have us believe. The whole antigen-antibody paradigm was a massive oversimplification. But as always in marketing, there's the KISS principle. No need to abandon a perfectly good theory just because it isn't true. Like the Germ Theory of Disease, the antigen-antibody model was a great teaching tool to substantiate the need for a ton of vaccines to be ramjetted into the bloodstream of mankind, from Pasteur till the end of time.

NATURAL IMMUNITY

happens only after recovering from the actual disease. Or at least being exposed to it. For example, on p. 1098 of the *Merck Manual* we find that for measles, **"... people born before 1956 are considered immune by virtue of prior infection."** [266] Natural immunity. With the actual disease, the organism has to pass through many of the body's natural immune defense systems in the nose, throat, and lungs before it ever gets as far as the bloodstream. It's likely that the organism slowly triggers many unknown biological events, essential in building true natural immunity, before it ever reaches the bloodstream.

Vaccination by direct injection makes the unproven assumption that the mere artificial stimulation of antibody production by the sudden presence of a foreign agent in the bloodstream is the whole story of immunity. Obviously it isn't; the need for booster shots proves that. Many studies have shown low antibody counts in vaccinated people. (Gunn, Fraser) [282, 16]

FOOLING MOTHER NATURE

Attenuated means half-killed. In vaccines the 'infectious agent' is weakened so that it is just below the threshold of being able to trigger an inflammatory response in 99.9% of people. By allowing the implantation of an attenuated virus or bacteria into the body, we have done something nature would never permit. We have violated the sanctity of the bloodstream. We have tricked the immune system into **not** mounting an all-out response to a foreign agent. If the microorganisms were not attenuated, the powers of the natural immune system would join together to repel and attack the invader.

Let's not forget – these aren't the original bugs associated with the disease they're using here, but rather manmade, lab versions of the original microbes.

Harvard Medical School's Dr. Richard Moskowitz explains that the way vaccines are evolved is to make them weaker and weaker, just to the point where they don't produce an immune response. The problem is, in this form, the altered microbes can penetrate far deeper into our tissues than would naturally have been possible. There they can become latent, hidden **allergens,** just waiting. Like a **slow virus**. Then when something triggers them into action, even years later, the stowaway microorganisms can manifest themselves in virtually any location or system of the body, causing dysfunction, chaos, degenerative disease, or even death. **But not from the original disease.** [103, 203]

That way no one can ever prove the vaccine was the cause of death – it's a beautiful thing.

Vaccination is a major detour from the path of human evolution. It took Nature a million years to come up with an immune system that would initiate an inflammatory response to these foreign agents. That's a survival mechanism. Herd immunity. Selection. Now suddenly in the past century, doctors are going to pretend they know enough to ignore aeons of natural wisdom?

VIRAL LOAD

Below we will see the problems with the toxic ingredients used in the manufacture of vaccines. But we must not forget that even if all these additives were eliminated from vaccines tomorrow, the biggest danger will remain as long as there are vaccines: viral load. That means the total accumulation of foreign virus and microorganisms that are introduced into the human bloodstream via vaccinations.

As you'll remember, a virus has the annoying talent of being able to splice itself into the DNA of a host cell. Taken together, the collective DNA of our race is known as the **human genome**. (Bishop) [217] Continuing to add more and more lab-altered versions of unknown foreign agents into our children's blood year after year is certain to be diluting the human genome. Such long-term change within our species is an entire field that **has never been studied.**

Looking at the 68 vaccines currently given to American schoolkids, there's no end in sight. Plans are being laid for dozens more vaccines, which will simply be tacked on, as with the new Adult Schedule. As each individual vaccine goes through the FDA 'approval' process, is there any consideration being given to the composite effect of the immense microbial load on a formative immune system? Shockingly, none whatsoever! Not by the CDC, the FDA, or the NIH. Want to talk about science? Consider the standard procedure when a child misses a vaccine day. What happens? They usually just wait until the next time, and do what? Right, give all the shots for both visits **on one day**. That could be as many as 15 vaccines at once! Any safety testing for this flagrantly unscientific common practice? None.

CELL LINES THAT CAN'T DIE

The use of continuous cell lines or **immortal strains** to maintain continuity of a vaccine year after year, standard within the industry since Jenner, has been extensively criticized. (Thya.[294])

A possible correlation is obvious between culturing cells lines that cannot die and the creation of cancerous tumors. (McReardon [157]) Groups of cells that don't die.

In his excellent text on vaccines, Tedd Koren [186] points out the sharp increase of **childhood cancers** that appeared between 1960 and 1980, when US vaccines doubled.

Cancer mortality in the US since vaccination began, 1902: [206, 304]

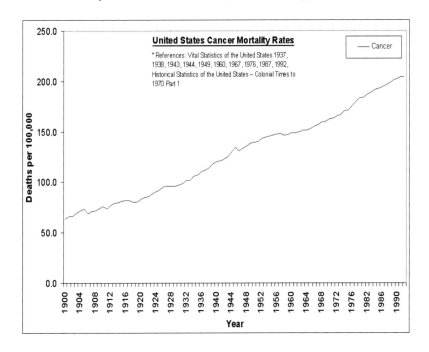

TRIPLE THREAT

Adverse reactions to vaccines can be divided into three types:

Immediate - like when the baby dies or else suffers some crisis in the first few hours or days after a shot

Latent - like when a toxin in the vaccine lodges itself in the brain causing a defect of brain architecture or a nerve disease that doesn't show up until years later.

Genome damage - where a foreign agent in the vaccine alters DNA, thereby causing cancer in a patient, or worse, having a general weakening effect on our collective DNA, the human genome.

The last of these is the worst. Viera uses the xerox analogy: as 16 billion injections a year access the DNA of human children, it's like making a copy of a copy of a copy, etc. The human genome is being diluted. The implications of such a trend on our species could hardly be more profound. [247]

THE RAT THEORY OF GARBAGE

The other problem is that the original theory was flawed: the bug attenuated in the vaccine wasn't the real **cause** of the original disease. Just like rats don't cause garbage, (Jensen, [237]) but are a result of untended garbage, germs don't cause disease. They're just seeking a congenial habitat. (Carrel [278]) They're the clean-up crew. Microbes are the evidence of disease, not the cause. Scavengers not predators.

Even Pasteur finally admitted that one, repudiating his own precious Germ Theory in one of the most quoted deathbed comments of all time:

> **"The terrain is everything; the germ is nothing."**   [202]

So here's the deal: for the love of money, we're going to legislate the following falsehoods as true:

1. a certain germ causes a certain disease

2. we'll give you immunity to that disease by injecting a weak version of the germ that doesn't cause the disease, directly into your bloodstream

NO LONG TERM STUDIES FOR VACCINE APPROVAL

In the U.S., there are almost never any long-term studies before a vaccine gets approved for mass use. H1N1 vaccine for example was approved after **6 weeks**. [47] Measles vaccine was approved after studies that only lasted **28 days**. (*Through a Glass* [147]) Chickenpox vaccine was approved after trials which lasted only **42 days**. [126] Hepatitis B vaccine was approved after **5 days**! [264] Nor is follow-up for long-term effectiveness of vaccines required. That's why the vaccines are always being altered and replaced – it's no metaphor to say our children are the lab rats.

IMMUNE RESPONSE VS. IMMUNITY

The whole shell game of vaccines can last only as long as people stay distracted from one central fact: the ability to produce an immune response does not by itself create immunity. Any toxic or poisonous stimulus may provoke some sort of immune reaction – some kind of inflammation, or fluxing out. So what? That is wholly separate from adding to the body's cumulative memory of how to defend against specific disease processes.

Vaccination is merely the artificial triggering of temporary responses to manmade pathogens. Immunity? Well, that's another foxhunt altogether.

Australian scientist Viera Scheibner, PhD states: [239]

'There is only one immunity, natural immunity, which is achieved by going through the infectious diseases of childhood.'

In 1888 French scientist Dr Xavier Raspail stated: "any antigen will produce a reaction and, more often than not, the immune system indicates its response in the form of antibodies. But their presence does not prove that they will protect, i.e. immunise." [302]

IMMUNITY: NATURAL VS. ARTIFICIAL

When a child gets a new disease, his newly forming immune system switches on. He may feel sick for several days, to one degree or another, but in the vast majority of cases, he is going to recover. If the body is allowed to figure out how to fight the disease on its own, without the added confusion and burden of powerful drugs and vaccines, the body will not be susceptible to that disease in the future, **for life**. Now it has an immunity to that disease - a memory of how to fight it. When the body acquires such memory on its own, with no drugs, we have **natural immunity.** The body now has a new, permanent weapon to protect itself from unfriendlies in the environment. This is why unvaccinated kids only get chickenpox once in their lives. The more weapons the body is allowed to create on its own, the less susceptible it will be to environmental stressors and diseases as an adult.

Natural immunity can be transferred from a mother to the fetus.

Natural immunity is the only true immunity. It happens after getting the disease or being exposed to the disease.

Artificial immunity, by contrast, means that the symptoms of the disease were artificially suppressed by means of drugs or **vaccines**. The nasal sprays and cough suppressants and anti-inflammatories allowed the foreign agent to get much deeper into the body than it otherwise might have gone, because the coughing and runny nose are basic clearing mechanisms to repel invaders. Doctors who pretend that the cough and the nasal congestion **are** the disease overlook the underlying cause.

"This suppression of symptoms prevents the body... from discharging what needs to come out..."   (James, p 42)   [199]

With vaccines, a manmade version of the presumed disease bug is injected into the bloodstream. The theory is that the body will produce antibodies to this weakened version, and ever after, those antibodies will be able to recognize and overwhelm the disease bugs if they ever show up again.

Such immunity is **artificial**, which really means inexact, because the vaccine is giving the body some sort of immunity not to the naturally occurring disease, but to a **mutant version** that chemists created in a lab.

Vaccines are the same for thousands and millions of doses. But each person's immune system and also the particular way a disease may occur in people - both these are unique. A flawed design from the get-go.

Artificial immunity cannot be passed from mother to fetus.

Artificial immunity is **temporary**. This is the reason for the unproven modern concept of **booster shots**.   (Murphy) [210]

Artificial immunity from vaccinations has created today's phenomenon of new **atypical forms** of the original disease appearing during adulthood, which can be much more serious and dangerous. As in adult measles, chickenpox, and shingles.

MASS VACCINATION - CREATING NEW DISEASES

No one ever talks about how these brand new **atypical** disease forms may be a threat to those who already have natural immunity, having got the original disease. Before mass vaccinations, the human species was building **herd immunity** to all the infectious diseases, to one degree or another. But that took 200,000 years. Those who got measles as a child and who now have lifetime immunity, may not be immune to the new manmade atypical adult forms of measles resulting from mass vaccination. Why not? Because the new form has only been around for about 30 years, whereas measles has been around for centuries. Just like superfluous antibiotics causing super-bugs, vaccination is creating new diseases.

Is that progress?

BOOSTERS

If the original vaccine conferred immunity, then why does the child need another shot 2 months later? What was the first one for? The fact is, **studies showing the efficacy of booster shots have never been done. For any vaccine**.

EVERYTHING IS YOU

Immunity is the body's ability to establish and maintain molecular identity. (James p105 [199] That means all your cells should look like you. They all came from the same DNA, right? Anything that promotes this uniformity brings health; whatever opposes the body's ability to maintain molecular identity brings disease. Understanding this simple principle explains why artificial immunity from vaccinations can't be long-term.

The whole process of creating a vaccine is to make some disease agent gradually weaker and weaker, until it is below the threshold of causing a reaction in 99.9% of children. That is, it's too weak for the body to recognize as foreign, and can penetrate far deeper into the body than nature would ever have allowed. The immune system DOES NOT get triggered the way it would by a foreign protein. We've tricked the body into **not responding**.

Such a process is outside the normal course of biological events; nothing like this ever occurs in nature. [203]

By contrast, the natural disease itself is strong enough to trigger the whole chain of normal immune responses.
Immunity cannot be forced upon the body. The body must

recognize the challenge of an actual foreign invader, and then be given the opportunity to put the pieces of the puzzle together all by itself, to figure out what combination of its own immune powers can recognize, surround, and overcome the foreign agent. This takes time and effort – **gentle, regular stimulation**. It may involve sickness. The process is far beyond the understanding of human science. But the result is lasting immunity – the only immunity.

HOW MANY VACCINATIONS?

Before 9/11 it was fairly easy to determine the number of mandated vaccines. The primary source for the vaccine Schedule is the CDC website. [26] But after 9/11, the Schedule began to change every few months, with new vaccines added and old ones removed, in an inexplicable fashion. To add to the confusion, the most recent trick is to have more than one Schedule, based on age category.

In the past it was always called the **Recommended Schedule for Childhood Immunization**, and it was from birth to 18 years. Then one day in 2008, The Childhood Schedule, The Adolescent Schedule, the Catch Up Schedule, and the **Adult Schedule** suddenly appeared on the CDC site, looking as though they had been there for 20 years. These charts are very difficult to read, and have many exceptions and overlaps. But their main effect is to obscure the skyrocketing number of total vaccines now being mandated for children. And dozens more for adults.

On the following pages we have the shocking schedule of the **68** Recommended Childhood Immunizations as of 2011 from the Centers for Disease Control. [26]

IMMUNIZATION SCHEDULE   2011

BIRTH:	hepatitis B	1 vaccine
1-2 MONTHS	hepatitis B	1 vaccine
2 MONTHS	Diphtheria-Pertussis-Tetanus Polio HiB PCV Rotateq	7 vaccines
4 MONTHS	Diphtheria-Pertussis-Tetanus Polio HiB PCV Rotateq	7 vaccines
6 MONTHS	Diphtheria-Pertussis-Tetanus PCV HiB Rotateq	6 vaccines
6 MONTHS - 18 YEARS	Influenza (yearly)	1 vaccine
6 - 18 MONTHS	Hepatitis B, Polio	2 vaccines
12-15 MONTHS	MMR HiB PCV Varicella	6 vaccines
12-23 MONTHS	Hepatitis A (twice)	2 vaccines
15-18 MONTHS	Diphtheria-Pertussis-Tetanus	3 vaccines

36 vaccines by 18 months of age

4 to 6 YEARS	Diphtheria-Pertussis-Tetanus MMR Polio Varicella	8 vaccines

11-12 YEARS   Tetanus /diphtheria /pertussis
HPV (3 doses)   MCV4   **7 vaccines**

68 TOTAL VACCINES
Source: Centers for Disease Control   www.cdc.gov [26]

The schedule underwent a major overhaul in early 2007. Since 9/11, changes are made much more frequently, sometimes only a few months apart. The total number was increased 3 separate times during 2007 alone. And again in 2008.

This list makes American children not only the most vaccinated children in the world - they are the most vaccinated group in the **history** of the world.   No other country on earth has such an aggressive program of vaccines.

Again, if a child misses a vaccine day, what happens the next time around? Right. All shots are given on the same day! Could be as many as 15 different vaccines! Any research proving this routine practice is safe? Absolutely none.

SET-UP FOR FUTURE VACCINES

The **High Risk Category**, the 2002 device that created a kind of back door to full approval for new experimentals, gracefully ensures a future of endless vaccines. Starting with the hysteria surrounding bioterrorism, we were set up for a whole string of new vaccines that could be quietly introduced at any time, just like Hep A, Rotateq and HPV were. Easy enough - just put them into the High Risk Category for a few months first. Then suddenly one day with no announcement whatsoever, poof! – suddenly they're whisked into the main Schedule. As if they'd been there forever…

Popping up just 4 short months after 9/11, this Category facilitates the administration of edicts allowed by the draconian Model Emergency Health Powers Act, Patriot Act, and the Homeland Security Act, presently the law of the land.   [166]

Such Fourth Reich legislation grants absolute powers to proclaim virtually any situation a terrorist emergency, and to decree that all or any part of the population must submit to whatever health measures are deemed necessary, including experimental vaccines.

Those who refuse may be fined, quarantined, prosecuted, imprisoned, or forced to submit, and property may be burned or confiscated.

Why not toss in the guillotine?

It seems unlikely that the provisions of legislation this extreme would ever be carried out, although versions of it are now the law of the land. But given these two options, Nazis-R-Us or Terrorists Might Pop Up Here And There, give me the threat of terrorism any day of the week. Haven't we seen how well they can protect us from anything?

HOW MANY ARE ENOUGH?

At 68 vaccines presently given to the most vaccinated children in the history of the world, you'd think the manufacturers would be content with the Golden Goose the way it is. They're not.

Legitimate scientific questions such as the overall effect of the total viral load from all these shots, the combinations of vaccines given in one shot, or on the same day - these concerns are never voiced, never funded for study. All we're concerned with is more, more, how much more, and how soon.

Look at this chart of total Mandated vaccines in recent years:

> 1980 20 vaccines
> 2003 40 vaccines
> 2004 53 vaccines
> 2005 58 vaccines
> 2006 63 vaccines
> 2011 68 vaccines

And that's just the children's vaccines.

THE NEW ADULT VACCINE SCHEDULE

What is far more unsettling than the above 68 is that suddenly in early 2008 an entire new era of vaccination was ushered in without a whisper of media coverage. In one quiet stroke the CDC just doubled the total number of vaccines recommended to Americans, with the introduction of the Adult Immunization Schedule, which is now recommending as many as **73 additional vaccines after the age of 18.** [26]

Didn't hear the evening newsreaders mention that one did you?

Suddenly out of the blue, after a century of vaccinating the American public, the CDC and their handlers decided that immunization isn't something that should be confined to childhood. No, no -- that leaves out the best marketing years of all: adulthood. For the past century, scientists have never claimed that vaccines confer lifetime immunity. Adult immunization was inevitable. Crossover marketing: booster shots for life! Why on earth didn't we think of this before? Double the American market, in one fell swoop.

Adult vaccine recommendation as of 2011:

TetanusDiphtheriaPertussis	**15**	
Human PapillomaVirus	**3**	
MeaslesMumpsRubella	**6**	
Varicella	**2**	
Influenza	**45**	
Prevnar	**1**	
Zoster	**1**	[26]

No other country on earth has an adult schedule of vaccines. No other country on earth recommends 150 vaccines to its citizens. The implications of this new policy cannot easily be apprehended. But it's safe to say that the cumulative detrimental effects from vaccines cited throughout this text essentially doubled for any Americans reckless enough to take part in the new adult experiment on the live population.

INFANTS ARE NOT MINIATURE ADULTS

Another idea that is never talked about is the size of an infant in comparison to the toxicity of a vaccine. From Dr Boyd Haley:

"A single vaccine given to a 6 pound newborn is the same as giving a 180-lb adult 30 vaccines on the same day." [133]

Treating the infant circulatory system like any other market, cavalierly applying sky's-the-limit corporate positioning principles, no one is asking the most fundamental question:

HOW MANY CAN THEY TAKE?

Hard on the heels of post 9/11 vaccine hysteria, with its provocative godknowswhat terrorist bioweapons about to be unleashed, we saw an astounding article in the Jan 2002 issue of the journal *Pediatrics*, that offered us a preview of science for the near future. On p 124 the authors reassure parents not to worry that their children are getting too many vaccines. It's OK because they've just found out that an infant can safely withstand **10,000** vaccines! Just by chance the article was authored by a member of the CDC Advisory Board, Paul 'For Profit' Offit.

Offit's prognostications helped encourage the total number of recommended vaccines to have **tripled** since 9/11.   [150]

INFANT MORTALITY WORLDWIDE

Do all these vaccines work? Are our children immune to all these diseases?

If vaccines really worked, shouldn't America be closer to the top of the list of infant mortality, instead of **#46**? [20] That means that the infants in 45 other countries of the world stand a better chance of survival to age 1 than ours do. And it's going in the wrong direction, because in 1997 we were #22! (UNICEF) [94]

At least **10,000** American babies mysteriously die each year with the catch-all **Sudden Infant Death Syndrome** (SIDS) diagnosis. That means the baby went to bed fine and woke up dead. Cause is always "unknown." Before mass vaccinations, the term didn't exist. (Mendelsohn)[241] The actual number is not being tracked. Viera Scheibner is the real expert on SIDS. Her life's work shows an unmistakable correlation with vaccines. [239]

The overall health of American children is abysmal: autoimmune disease, asthma, allergies, and worse, the very infectious diseases for which they were vaccinated - all are on the rise:

"There is a growing suspicion that immunization against relative harmless childhood diseases may be responsible for the dramatic increase in autoimmune diseases since mass inoculations were introduced... cancer, leukemia, rheumatoid arthritis, MS, Lou Gehrig's disease, lupus, and Guillain-Barre' syndrome."
                                                      - p 232, *How To Raise...* [241]

Dr. Mendelsohn wrote this 25 years ago. Are these diseases disappearing? How did 'autoimmune' become a household word? What about chronic fatigue, autism, mysterious chronic allergies and arthritic problems that are affecting increasingly younger people in the past few years? Are more or less kids these days walking through school corridors sniffing inhalers? For spending over $2 trillion annually on health care, our health doesn't seem to reflect it.

INFANT HOSPICE

In July 2002 a shocking story appeared in the news that drew very little attention: it seems the National Institutes of Health, which is the government agency that funds most medical research in the US, had just put aside **$2.5 million** to create end of life care for infants. Now let's stop and think for a minute what that means. Like with hospice care for people who are dying of cancer and other terminal illnesses, our government had just determined that so many infants are dying slow deaths from diseases, that it is now necessary to create a program to help them shuffle loose the mortal coil. The number? **53,000 infants per year**, dying of terminal diseases. Not accidental deaths, mind you -- terminal diseases they acquired since birth. This is a staggering figure - nearly the total number of Americans who died in the Vietnam War. Or at Gettysburg. Except it's happening **every year**. [153]   To infants.

HERD IMMUNITY: THE TRUE STATISTICS

Medical statistician Michael Alderson does a thorough job of showing how infectious diseases had run their course through the human race before mass 'immunizations' ever came upon the scene. Looking at the data, it is patently clear that infectious diseases would have largely disappeared without any vaccines. Just as they did all through history.

We always hear about how vaccination has saved us from infectious diseases, etc. Or we hear from the anti-vaccine crowd how infectious diseases have resolved on their own during the last century, without the help of vaccines. But how often does either side offer proof?

So, which is it? Here is the documentation that settles the question once and for all:

Figure 1. DEATHS PER 100,000, U.S.

	Diphtheria	Pertussis	Measles	Influenza
1900	40.3	12.2	13.3	202.2
1910	21.1	11.6	12.4	155.9
1920	15.3	12.5	8.8	207.3
1930	4.9	4.8	3.2	102.5
1940	1.1	2.2	.5	70.3
1945	1.2	1.3	.2	51.6
1950	.3	.7	.3	31.3
1955	.1	.3	.2	27.1
1960	0	.1	.2	37.3
1970	0	0	0	30.9

Source: *Historical Statistics* [206] This government reference can be found in any library.

On the next page is a chart showing death incidence every 5 years for each disease.

Underlined number in chart below indicates the approximate advent of vaccine. - (*International Mortality Statistics*, pp. 163-189, 313, Michael Alderson [213])

Figure 2.   USA DEATHS

Year	POLIO	DIPHTHERIA	PERTUSSIS
1901		48,839	33,094
1906-		28,225	26,436
1911-		20,350	20,285
1916-		15,623	21,382
1921-	7229	12,267	14,724
1926-	6038	7074	13,047
1931-	4545	4388	9850
1936-	3666	2189	6809
1941-	3539	1135	4399
1946-	3799	<u>467</u>	<u>1460</u>
1951-	3826	125	558
1956-	<u>1604</u>	45	206
1961-	1076	22	82
1966-	928	15	32
1971-75	0	12	122

Year	TETANUS	MEASLES	INFLUENZA
1901	28,065	11,956	15,496
1906-	16,318	10,837	10,109
1911-	11,503	7615	7086
1916-	8596	7926	54,283
1921-	7818	4919	13,673
1926-	6040	3994	17,602
1931-	4709	2957	11,191
1936-	3275	1238	8449
1941-	2384	1013	4366
1946-	<u>1697</u>	469	1736
1951-	1093	268	1178
1956-	788	203	938
1961-	550	162	553
1966-	282	44	633
1971-75	122	<u>17</u>	491

So as we see the natural decline of diseases, next we must ask when did the individual vaccines come in?

Here are the exact years:

Disease	Vaccinations
polio............................	1954
smallpox......................	1902
diphtheria....................	mid 1940s
pertussis......................	mid 1940s
tetanus.........................	mid 1940s
MMR........................	1978
hemophilus b............	1985
hepatitis B...................	1991
chickenpox	1995
PCV	2002
influenza	2005

Take a minute and go back and look at these last charts, until it dawns on you that these diseases were on their way out long before vaccines took the headlines.

Here's an independent opinion from a source with no medical axe to grind:

"...the death rate of diphtheria, measles, and whooping cough declined 95 percent among children from 1911 to 1945, before the mass immunization programs started in the United States."   [263] Metropolitan Life Insurance

BIOSTATISTICS: DOING ANYTHING WITH NUMBERS

The above data are unadorned statistics from valid sources available in any library. Try digging them up on your own – this plain evidence is buried.

A favorite trick of op-ed writers and publications documenting the magnificent success of vaccines is to make up numbers or charts without citing sources. Such statements are meaningless. Where did the figures come from? A psychic relative? An apparition? If you can't look something up, never believe anyone's "statistics." Especially if the sentence starts out with the words "recent studies have shown..." A stock phrase of junk science.

THE SCUM ALSO RISES

When it comes to the volatile area of Political Immunology, reporting deaths and bad reactions from vaccination has been a very sensitive area, right from the start. Obviously those selling vaccines are not going to want to advertise their failures - that's just business. But creating false data and omitting reports of adverse reactions, that gets into a whole other area of fraud and misrepresentation.

The other smokescreen commonly used by statisticians and writers is the Too Much Data trick. They'll divide the raw data up into so many subgroups, like age, sex, and race, that the main idea gets obscured. In this way, simple facts like the per capita increase in US cancer deaths in the past 50 years, or the natural decline in deaths from diseases before vaccinations came out - things like this get conveniently lost. (Yiamouyiannis, p 78) [214]

Most people don't read medical journals and books;   they skim a few e-zines, and form their opinions from a few bytes of what they find there. Pop media tend to support the agenda of their main advertisers - the drug companies.

In the pediatrics profession, it's much simpler. Adverse reactions simply don't get reported. In fact, they are routinely met with immediate denial. It's just basic economics. Vaccinations are the bread and butter of pediatricians - the Well Baby programs. Anything that undermines people's confidence in vaccines threatens the profession's livelihood. Not to mention legal threats of malpractice.

REPORTING ADVERSE REACTIONS

As far as physicians' responsibility for reporting adverse reactions, feature this: mass vaccination programs have been rolling in the US since 1902. But until 1991, there was "no central record keeping agency in the U.S. to which physicians could report vaccine reactions." (p 88 [227]) In 1991, the VAERS (Vaccine Adverse Effect Reporting System) was set up in the US.

The NCVIA was the 1986 law signed by Ronald Reagan to let drug companies off the hook when children died from side effects by decreeing: "no vaccine manufacturer shall be liable ... for damages arising from a vaccine-related injury or death." ([248] p.499)

Before 1991, any statement about the safety of vaccines was meaningless because there was no central reporting agency keeping track of adverse reactions! Everyone was saying how safe vaccinations were, but how would they know if no one were tracking the reactions? If a kid dropped dead 5 minutes after a vaccine, no one kept count of it before 1991. So we have no idea of the actual numbers. Then as now, the majority of doctors simply don't report vaccines reactions. The FDA estimates that doctors only report 10% of adverse reactions to vaccinations. (Orient, Null) [190, 220, 240]

One big reason why only 10% are reported is that no one wants to admit liability. Most doctors have the Orwellian programming to think that if they report a true adverse reaction, it will undermine public confidence in vaccination!

Although no studies support it, the 10% figure has been arbitrarily selected and appears consistently in CDC and FDA literature when estimating the number of reactions that get reported. A study by NVIC of New York doctors found only **2%** of doctors admit that they report adverse reactions. It's entirely possible that only 1% of adverse reactions to vaccines ever get reported to VICP. [261]

HOW MANY REACTIONS REALLY?

It is almost impossible to decipher the charts appearing on the VICP site and calculate the total number of deaths and reactions from vaccines. Obviously that is the intent. By 2004, over **200,000 adverse event reports** were recorded in the VICP database following more than one billion doses of more than 30 different types of vaccines administered as part of the U.S. National Immunization Program. (Geier, [118] [35]) If this represented only 10% of actual, that's 2 million serious vaccine reactions since 1991.

Now if the true figure is really 1% of actual reactions, as FDA Commissioner Kessler stated it was [310], that means that there could have been **20 million** serious adverse reactions to vaccines since 1991, involving either death, permanent injury or hospitalization. Such an epidemic could actually be in place in the US at the present time and no one is even clocking it!

Don't we all know at least one vaccine-injured child?

TIME LIMIT

According to VICP rules, there are very strict criteria for reporting an adverse reaction to vaccines. One of these is the arbitrary time limit for filing:

"In the case of an injury, the claim must be filed **within 36 months** after the first symptoms appeared" (NVIC [261])

But many reactions don't show up until much later in life: the latent organic type of injury, from toxic adjuvants, causing defects in the formative brain tissues of the infant. Anything later than 36 months doesn't count, and can never be compensated.

RECAP:

- Some 68 vaccines are mandated in this country for children

- No one knows how many thousands have died or suffered adverse reactions from the vaccines, since there was no reporting agency in place until 1991.

- The drug companies are exempt from prosecution

- Less than 10% of actual ill effects are reported

- There is no follow-up on the reported cases, some of which involve death or permanent neurological damage.

- Compensation for vaccine injuries is borne by the taxpayers

Yes, yes, it's staggering.

POURCYROUS STUDY: PEER REVIEW PROVES VACCINES CAUSE BRAIN INJURY

The next time your hear someone reciting the rote mantra about how there's no proof vaccines cause brain injury, stop them in mid-sentence with this study.

One of the most credible sources proving vaccines cause brain injuries in babies is certainly the landmark **Pourcyrous study** on brain inflammation following vaccines.   [251]

It was a very thorough University of Tennessee study of **239 premature infants**, measuring injuries from both single and multiple vaccines.

They looked at 2 things: **C-reactive protein** and evaluation of **cardiopulmonary function.**

C-reactive protein is a blood value, high levels of which indicate inflammation. In this case, of the brain.

Results: **Among preemies getting a single vaccine shot: 70% had high CRP.**

Preemies who got multiple vaccines: 85% had high CRP.

Fully **16% had cardiopulmonary events within 48 hours,** including **apnea** and **bradycardia**. In a preemie, these effects are potentially fatal, of course.

Brain hemorrhages occurred in 17% of those with single vaccines, and in 24% getting multiple vaccines.

As expected, the most dangerous vaccine was DPT. Multiple vaccines included Hepatitis B, polio, DPT, H. influenzae, and Prevnar.

What kind of "scientist" would it take to even conduct a study like this in the first place on the fragile systems of premature infants? And if these dangerous results are so high at this age, how much better results could we expect just a few weeks later when most babies start getting multiple vaccines?

What are we doing? How smart or how dumb do you have to be – we're this careless with the most delicate medium in the universe: the infant's brain neurology? You can bet these geniuses aren't experimenting with their own children.

Here's how the conclusion of this study evaluates its own data:

"In a minority of infants immunized, cardiorespiratory events were associated with presumed need for intervention"

A minority? 17% is a pretty high minority especially if you're talking about the chances of your own infant dying from slowed heart rate and cessation of breathing! And for what? The value of vaccines has never been clearly demonstrated, never proven in an independent controlled risk/benefit analysis. In other words, we don't know if they work or not. But we're positive they can kill. "Presumed need for intervention"? Like what? Drugs? Intensive care? How about omitting the danger itself?

As a parent, wouldn't it be important to know that your child stands a 17% chance of a breathing crisis as the result of a vaccine? Or a 24% chance of brain hemorrhage with multiple vaccines, which multiples routinely begin at 2 months of age, with 7 vaccines on one day? Is the pediatrician going to tell the parents about these studies? Isn't this level of danger worth knowing about?

What are we doing to our kids?

THE PEANUT ALLERGY EPIDEMIC

Have you ever wondered why so many kids these days are allergic to peanuts? Where did this allergy come from all of a sudden?

Before 1900, violent reactions to peanuts were unheard of. Today over a million children in this country are allergic to peanuts.

What happened? Why is everybody buying EpiPens now?

Looking at all the problems with vaccines during the past decade, just a superficial awareness is enough to raise the suspicion that vaccines have some role in the appearance of any novel allergy among children.

But reactions to peanuts are not just another allergy. Peanut allergy has suddenly emerged as the **#1 cause of death from food reactions**, ([16] p 114) being in a category of allergens able to cause

anaphylaxis. This condition includes asthma attack, shock, respiratory failure, and even death. Primarily among children.

New research in Heather Fraser's 2011 book *The Peanut Allergy Epidemic* defines the vaccine connection much more specifically. We now learn that a class of vaccine ingredients - **excipients** - is more than a likely suspect in what may accurately be termed an epidemic.

But let's back up a little. We have to look at both vaccines and antibiotics in recent history, and the physical changes that the ingredients in these brand new medicines introduced into the blood of children.

SHOCK REACTIONS

Before 1900, anaphylactic shock was virtually unknown. The syndrome of sudden collapse, respiratory distress, convulsions, and sometimes death did not exist until smallpox vaccinators switched from the lancet to the hypodermic needle. That transformation was essentially complete by the turn of the century in the western world.

Right at that time a new disease called **Serum Sickness** began to claim thousands of children. A variety of symptoms, including shock and death, could suddenly result following an injection of vaccine. Instead of covering it up, the connection with vaccine shots was well recognized and documented in the medical literature of the day. Serum Sickness was the first mass allergenic phenomenon in history.

Serum Sickness was a known consequence of vaccinations. Indeed, the entire field of modern allergy has evolved from the early study of Serum Sickness following vaccination.

"Mass allergic phenomena first emerged as a side effect of late 19th century technology – vaccination with a hypodermic syringe." Fraser, p 67 [16]

ANAPHYLAXIS

A Nobel laureate of the early 1900s - **Dr Charles Richet** - was the man who coined the term **anaphylaxis**. [326] His field was the reactions that some people seemed to have to certain foods. Richet found that with food allergies the reaction came on as the result of **intact proteins** in the food having bypassed the digestive system and making their way intact into the blood, via Leaky Gut. Foreign protein in the blood, of course, is a universal trigger for allergic reaction, not just in man but in all animals.

But Richet noted that in the severe cases, food anaphylaxis did not happen just by eating a food. That would simply be food poisoning.

Food anaphylaxis is altogether different. This sudden, violent reaction requires an initial sensitivity involving injection of some sort, followed by a later ingestion of the sensitized food. Get the shot, then later eat the food.

The initial exposure created the **hypersensitivity**. The second exposure would be the violent, perhaps fatal, physical event.

Richet regarded anaphylaxis as part of **Natural Selection**, nature's command to keep the proteins of different species separate from each other:

> "Anaphylaxis, perhaps a sorry matter for the individual, is necessary to the species, often to the detriment of the individual. The individual may perish, it does not matter. The species must at any time keep its organic integrity intact.

Anaphylaxis defends the species against the peril of adulteration.

> "We … can never receive other proteins into the blood than those that have been modified by digestive juices.

> "Every time alien protein penetrates …, the organism suffers and becomes resistant. This resistance lies in increased sensitivity, a sort of revolt against the second injection, which would be fatal. At the first injection, the organism was taken by surprise and did not resist. At the second injection, the organism mans its defences and answers by the anaphylactic shock.

> "Seen in these terms, anaphylaxis is an universal defence mechanism against the penetration of heterogenous substances in the blood, whence they cannot be eliminated."

Richet's early work around 1900 was primarily with eggs, meat, milk and diphtheria proteins. Not peanuts, and not vaccines. The value of Richet's research with reactive foods was to teach us the pathways of allergic sensitivity to foreign proteins, leading to anaphylaxis, how that had to take place.

PENICILLIN AND EXCIPIENTS

Next up was penicillin, which became popular in the 1940s. It was soon found that additives called **excipients** were necessary to prolong the effect of the injected antibiotic. The excipients would act as carrier molecules. Without excipients, the penicillin would only last about 2 hours. Refined oils worked best, acting as time-release capsules for the antibiotic. Peanut oil became the favorite, increasing penicillin's activity to about 48 hours.

As allergy to penicillin became common, it was recognized as a sensitivity to the excipient oils. ([16], p 94) To the present day a standard screening test in all clinics is always to ask a new patient about possible allergies to antibiotics. That's what the antibiotic allergy is - a sensitivity to the excipients.

By 1953 as many as **12% of the population** was allergic to penicillin. There were many fatal reactions once penicillin became widespread. But considering the upside with bacterial infections, it was still considered a worthwhile risk.

By 1950 antibiotics were being given out like M&Ms. Soldiers, children, anybody with any illness, not just bacterial. Despite Fleming's severe warnings against prophylactic antibiotics, antibiotics were given indiscriminately as the new wonder drug. Just in case anything. Only then, in the 1950s, did peanut allergy begin to occur, even though Americans had been eating peanuts for well over a century. Remember - just eating peanuts cannot cause peanut allergy. Unless they are allowed to become moldy of course, in which case aflatoxins are released. But that's really not a peanut allergy per se.

But even when peanut allergy did appear, the number of cases was fairly small and it wasn't even considered worthy of study.

PEANUT OILS IN VACCINES

The change came with **vaccines**. Peanut oils were introduced as vaccine excipients in the mid 1960s. By 1980 they had become the preferred excipient.

They were considered **adjuvants** - substances able to increase reactivity to the vaccine. This reinforced the **Adjuvant Myth**: the illusion that immune response is the same as immunity [327]: the pretense being that the stronger the allergic response to the vaccine, the greater will be the immunity that is conferred.

The first study of peanut allergies was not undertaken until 1973. It was a study of peanut excipients in vaccines. Soon afterwards, as a result of that study, manufacturers were no longer required to disclose all the ingredients in vaccines.

What is listed today in the *Physicians Desk Reference* in each vaccine section is not the full formula. Suddenly that detailed information was proprietary: the manufacturers must be protected. They only had to describe the formula in general.

Why was peanut allergy so violent? The famous Maurice Hilleman found that even the most refined peanut oils still contained some traces of **intact peanut proteins**. [16] This was the reason doctors were directed to inject vaccines intramuscular rather than intravenous - a greater chance of absorption of intact proteins, less chance of reaction.

But that obviously wasn't enough to prevent sensitivity. The fundamental law of nature always applies: no intact proteins in the body. 60 million years of Natural Selection didn't create the mammalian immune system for nothing. Put intact proteins, peanut or whatever, for any imagined reason into the human system and the inflammatory response will fire.

PEANUT EPIDEMIC BEGINS

Although peanut allergies became fairly common during the 1980s, it wasn't until the early 1990s when there was a sudden surge of children reacting to peanuts. Then the true epidemic appeared.

The Mandated Schedule of vaccines for children doubled from the 80s to the 90s:

1980   20 vaccines
1995   40 vaccines
2011   68 vaccines

It would be imprudent enough to feed peanuts to a newborn since their digestive system is largely unformed. But this is much worse - injecting intact proteins directly into the infant's blood. In 36 vaccines before the age of 18 months.

As vaccines doubled between the 1980s and the 1990s, thousands of kids were now exhibiting peanut sensitivities, with many violent reactions, sometimes fatal.

Following the next enormous increase in vaccines on the Mandated Schedule after 9/11 whereby the total shot up to 68 recommended vaccines, peanut allergy soon reached epidemic proportions: a **million children: 1.5% of them**. [16] These numbers fit the true definition of epidemic even though that word has never been used in mainstream literature with respect to peanut allergy, except in

Fraser's book.

This is another example of how vaccines specifically suppress the normal immune system. Those children most prone to allergy and hypersensitivity may be those who are the slowest to develop the ability to identify and clear poisons.

Many researchers, not only Fraser, could see very clearly that

   "The peanut allergy epidemic in children was precipitated by childhood injections."   ([16], p106)

But with the new research impugning vaccines, the medical profession will do what they always must do - bury it. Protect the companies. So no money will be ever allocated from NIH to study the obvious connection between vaccine excipients and peanut allergy. That cannot happen, primarily because it would require a **control group** - an unvaccinated population. And that is the Unspoken Forbidden. Same line of reasoning that has prevented Wakefield's work from ever being replicated in a mainstream US clinical study. No unvaccinated populations. Which actually means no studies whose outcome could possibly implicate vaccines as a source of disease or immunosuppression. Vaccines as a cause of an allergy epidemic? Impossible. Let's definitely not study it.

Instead let's spend the next 20 years looking for the Genetic Link to the childhood peanut allergy epidemic...

In such a flawed system, any pretense of true clinical science is fatally handicapped of course: we are looking for the truth, wherever our studies shall take us, except for this, and this, and oh yes, this.

Let's briefly evaluate some of the current vaccines being given. Now this may seem tedious, like too much information. But if you have a child you are about to vaccinate, can you really be making an informed decision when the sole source of your information comes from those making their living by selling shots? Take an evening away from TV here and inform yourself.

POLIOMYELITIS

Polio no longer exists in the Western world in its wild state. The only source of poliomyelitis since 1979 have been from the polio vaccine. (*Vaccine Guide* p 108 [215]) "The risk of acquiring wild polio in the US is zero."

A viral infection of the grey matter of the spinal cord, poliomyelitis in its natural state was never such a killer, even before vaccines came out. 90% of those who carried the polio virus never had any symptoms. (Burnet, p 93) [201] And only a fraction of 1% of cases ended up with long term paralysis. {215], p 108]

It is very doubtful that the polio vaccine was itself responsible for the decline of polio in the U.S. As we saw above in Figure 2, many researchers show how that decline was happening anyway. [213]

The sharp dropoff in polio cases reported on Alderson's statistics chart above is due to the radical change in the way polio cases were reported rather than to the effect of the vaccine itself. A complete explanation of this trick reporting can be found on p.109 of Neustaedter's *The Vaccine Guide*, [215] where the testimony of Dr. Bernard Greenberg, a government biostatistician, is quoted. To make a long story short, doctors over-reported polio before 1954, and under-reported it afterwards. Politics. They were motivated to show that the vaccine worked. Vaccination Fever, following on the coattails of the Golden Age of Antibiotics in the 1950s. Better living through chemistry.

From Dr Herbert Shelton,   (*Hygienic Care of Children*) :

"The apparent disappearance of polio was brought about by clever juggling. Before the Salk vaccine was introduced, thousands of cases of polio were diagnosed each year in children who had no polio.

"After the introduction of the vaccine, these cases were no longer diagnosed as polio. This automatically appeared to reduce the cases to a near vanishing point."   [233]

A little problem occurred in 1955 with some of the early lots of Salk polio vaccine. Some 80 children immediately got polio from the vaccine, and they spread it to at least another 120 kids. **Three of the victims died and 75% were paralyzed**. ([248], p 487)

What is certain is that polio is gone, but not because of the polio vaccine. The inventor of the vaccine, Jonas Salk himself testified in 1977 that the few cases of polio we now see in the U.S. are the result of using the polio vaccine rather than the result of the disease itself. (*Science Abstracts* **4 Apr 1977**)   [270]

Even the CDC also admits that **all cases of polio in the U.S. after 1979 have been caused by the vaccine**, not the disease! [212] p 568.

You parents checking this out? If the only cases of polio in America in the past 40 years are caused by the vaccine itself, why are we still vaccinating? With 4 shots?

Wouldn't be so bad if the vaccine were harmless. But there are two little complications that came with this "harmless" vaccine:

- the polio vaccine was "stabilized" with neurotoxins like mercury and formaldehyde
- the original polio vaccine contained the **SV-40** monkey virus

The first of these is beyond controversy. The manufacturers admitted it. (*Physicians' Desk Reference* [244])

Mercury, as we all know, is a metabolic poison, damaging brain, kidneys, and bone marrow. (Widman's, p.691; Bernard [207, 180]) Formaldehyde, used in embalming, is a known carcinogen.

The second of these complications, the contamination of polio vaccine with SV-40, bears elaboration.

50,000 MONKEYS

were slaughtered in the 60s in order to make the Salk vaccine for polio. (James, p166) [199] Tens of thousands of rhesus monkeys had been killed since 1952 to provide kidneys on which to culture the vaccine. (*PDR*, 1998 p 2131) [244] Looking at the statistics of polio during the past century (Figure 2 above), many researchers, including the inventor himself, later felt the polio vaccine was unnecessary, because by 1954 the disease was obviously winding itself down throughout our species.

Looking at a 1963 issue of *Science Digest* shows that in the 1950s a monkey virus named **SV-40** was "unwittingly put into hundreds of thousands, if not millions, of doses of Salk vaccine." (Snider) [218] And where did this happen? Africa. (Curtis, p1259) [219]   Some **98**

million doses of the SV contaminated polio vaccine were given to American children between 1955 and 1963. [173]

Horowitz shows that anyone who got polio vaccine prior to 1964 is probably carrying SV-40.   ([248] p. 493)

Later research linked SV-40 with cancer as well.   In Mar 02, scientists at University of Texas and at Baylor independently found the same high correlation (43%) between SV-40 and **non-Hodgkins lymphoma**, the fifth most common cancer in the US. (Beil) [167]

Leading scientist Michele Carbone MD: "... there are **more than 70 papers from 60 different laboratories that have confirmed the association of SV-40 with human ... bone and brain tumors.**" [122]

Jonas Salk's polio vaccine only lasted for 17 months because of all the deaths and paralysis it caused. Its replacement was the Sabin oral vaccine. Here's what Albert Sabin, MD, the inventor of that vaccine, had to say 30 years later:

   "Official data has shown that the large scale vaccinations undertaken in the US have failed to obtain any significant improvement of the diseases for which they were supposed to provide immunization. In essence it was and is a failure. " [275]

DISEASE FROM VACCINE

Polio vaccine is still unsafe today. In the Caribbean during 2002 there were 21 cases of polio and 2 deaths caused by the oral polio vaccine. [148, 144] The **vaccine itself has created a new disease,** capable of spreading from patient to patient, according to the CDC. [168] A CDC scientist, Olin Kew tells us that in this case:

"...the virus, originating in the vaccine ...had undergone a series of genetic mutations .., had reverted to a virulent form and caused the very disease it was meant to prevent."   [144]

The *Wall Street Journal* reported:

"Scientists had long speculated that the virus contained in the vaccine might re-emerge ... in a virulent form. But this had never been seen ...until Kew analyzed the changes in the Hispaniola bug....they saw the alarming manner in which the virus had 'back-mutated.' " [148]

BACKWATER VACCINE DUMPS

Hostility against US vaccine programs is becoming more and more evident in Third World places, who grasp the true politics of being the market for the First World's drug throwaways. [115] In Pakistan during much of 2008, fighting broke out among groups who were resisting mandatory polio shots from UNICEF [72], seeing vaccination as a genocidal effort. Difficult to justify trying to vaccinate half a million people in an area with only 32 cases of polio in all of 2007, especially with the vaccine's track record of fatal reactions.

Polio vaccine is clearly perpetuating a disease that would have disappeared completely on its own by now.

DPT – THE MOST TOXIC OF ALL

Next we have the famous DPT triple-shot cocktail - **diphtheria, pertussis, and tetanus**, all in one shot.   Let's briefly look at each disease:

DIPHTHERIA

Diphtheria, which means 'grey membrane,' was an old-time disease in which infection of the tongue and throat formed a grey membrane which in advanced cases could actually choke the victim to death.

Like polio and smallpox, diphtheria is a disease of the past, seen in conditions of overcrowding, lack of sanitation, and bad hygiene. It is no longer a risk today; Mendelsohn said there's about as much chance of dying from a cobra bite as from diphtheria. (*How To*, (p.245). [241]

In 2001, there were only **2 cases** in the entire US! [117] CDC cites no reported cases since 2005 in the US! [8] And yet millions are vaccinated endlessly for this defunct disease.   Again, Fig. 2 illustrates how diphtheria was responding to improvements in nutrition, water supply, and sanitation long before the vaccine became popular in the mid 1940s.

Does diphtheria vaccine work? Mendelsohn cites the 1969 Chicago diphtheria "epidemic" of 16 deaths. Some epidemic.

Nine of the 16 had been vaccinated! By the time the diphtheria vaccination was common in only half the states, there was no difference in incidence between the vaccinated states and the unvaccinated. Furthermore the vaccine has long been unnecessary because for years now this bacterial disease can be easily treated with **erythromycin**, a common antibiotic. No need for the vaccine. [266]

Although reports of adverse reactions from diphtheria shots have not piled up in the thousands the way they have for pertussis vaccine, the fact remains that no long-term studies of the diphtheria vaccine's effects have ever been carried out. Bottom line: there is no medical reason whatsoever to maintain diphtheria vaccination in this country.

Why are kids getting 5 doses of it then?

PERTUSSIS

Now we shall learn the meaning of lethal injection.

Pertussis is the medical term for **whooping cough**, a harsh disease that killed many infants in centuries past. The opportunistic agent was a bacterium, *B. pertussis*, airborne, invading the upper respiratory tract. With violent coughing so deep that all air was expelled, the desperate inhaling to refill the empty lungs would often make the victim give out the characteristic "whooping" sound. Some babies fractured ribs from the effort, and sometimes died from exhaustion.

Like other infectious diseases, pertussis favored crowded, unsanitary cities in both Europe and America. Many cities had famous epidemics which killed tens of thousands: Paris in 1578, Rome in 1695, London in the late 1850s. Whooping cough would commonly set up a secondary infection, usually pneumonia, which could then overtake the weakened patient. (p 5 [227])

Whooping cough was a disease of poverty, malnutrition, unsafe water, poor hygiene, and overcrowding. As conditions were gradually improved in the cities of Europe and America, infectious diseases declined dramatically, as Fig. 2 above shows. With pertussis, this chart is critical in understanding the minor role that vaccinations really played. Scottish researcher Dr. Gordon Stewart points out that pertussis was 80% resolved by the time any vaccines appeared. [235] In America, it was closer to 95%. [123]

Then, why the big push to mandate a vaccine for a disease that was almost gone? The usual reason.

Pertussis is the most controversial of American vaccines.

The only safety testing that has ever been done on the pertussis vaccine in the past 50 years is something called the **Mouse Weight Gain Test.** In the 1940s the "scientists" injected the vaccine to be tested into the stomachs of baby mice. If the mice continue to gain weight and didn't die right away, it was assumed the vaccine was safe and effective for humans. That's it! Not making this up. (Coulter, p11) [227] But this is not a vaccine for mice; it's for mass inoculation into the human population - American children.

The fact that hundreds of children have died and thousands more have reported adverse reactions from the pertussis component has not been cause enough to re-evaluate DPT.

WHY IS DPT A TRIPLE?

With no safety testing, a researcher named Pearl Kendrick in 1942 hit on the idea that the pertussis vaccine could simply be added to the diphtheria and tetanus vaccines, for the doctor's convenience. [238] **Trivalent**: 3 vaccines together. Sometimes when vaccines are mixed together, one activates the others and makes them more potent. And therefore more dangerous. **Viral interference** is the term. [271] So you'd think the combination of the three vaccines would have to be tested together, right?

The problem is, the three vaccines were never tested together before they were released on the market! Nor have they have been. (Wakefield) [271]

In the mid-1940s the pertussis vaccine was licensed and DPT became the standard version. The three vaccines were just mixed together, without considering the possible increased risk to infants. This statement is borne out by the history of documented adverse reactions to the DPT cocktail which do not occur with the DT vaccine alone. (Cody) [229] It is undisputed that the pertussis component of the vaccine is the main cause of adverse reactions.

THE UNDYING MYTHOLOGY OF TETANUS

This disease is said to be caused by an anaerobic bacillus called *Clostridium tetani*. Puncture wounds favor anaerobics - no oxygen in there. Here again, the disease seeks out those with the weakest immune systems – the starving, druggies, those in unhygienic surroundings... (*Merck Manual* p 1176). [266]

Merck puts the death rate at 50% for those who actually get the disease, although where that figure came from is anybody's guess. Death from tetanus is not that much fun, however - the muscles of the jaw, the back, and the diaphragm may go into unremitting spasm, choking the person, after a few days.

The thing is, it's gone. Referring again to Figure 2 above, we see the incidence of tetanus had almost completely disappeared by the time vaccines became popular. Tetanus vaccine has been a part of mass inoculation since the 1940s. It's the T of DPT. Since the

1950s, a child received DPT shots by the time he is 18 months old. Ever after that for life any time anyone steps on a nail or gets a minor cut, tetanus "boosters" are routinely given. But what sense does it make to pretend to cure a disease that is caused by a puncture wound which may have the remotest possibility of containing *Clostridium* by giving the person another puncture wound that definitely contains *Clostridium*, or its byproducts?

It's one thing to claim that the vaccine could confer immunity before the injury happened. But to pretend a shot could immunize someone after the infection has occurred trespasses into the realm of superstition. **No manufacturer has ever claimed curative power for any vaccine**. They're preventatives, remember? That's the whole basis of immunology.

As for tetanus boosters, Mendelsohn doubts the necessity any more often than every 40 years. (*How To*, p 195) [241]

A brilliant article was written by disease expert Dr Alec Burton in 1995. [305] Citing all his references, Burton discloses one hidden fact after another about the tetanus mythology:

Clostridium is everywhere: in the mouth, GI tract, and skin of healthy people, on clothing, in house dust. And yet tetanus is a rare disease. The bacilli were found in 20% of war wounds without any tetanus resulting. In 50% of actual tetanus cases no bacilli were found. *Clostridium* was shown to be harmless in pure culture. There is no evidence that tetanus vaccine prevents tetanus, nor has there ever been. But the vaccine has been shown to cause severe reactions, including death.   [305]

Again, no scientists claim curative value after being infected with

Clostridium. Nor do any suggest that a subsequent vaccine would prevent the development of tetanus. Think about it: if you have a disease process already going on, how could adding more of the pathogen or its toxoids to your blood possibly help you? That dog don't hunt. Pure science fiction. Only the clinics who actually give the shots would dare such a pretense. Point-of-sale closing technique.

We must violate the human bloodstream only when overwhelming proof indicates the necessity, instead of shooting kids up with a vaccine whose value has not been determined. Especially when the very act of vaccination is a puncture wound!

"Although not in the vaccine itself, this organism is an opportunist in any wound, and tetanus following vaccination is always to be feared." (S.Thomas) [316]

How did the conventional wisdom of tetanus shots from a dirty rusty nail outdoors where *Clostridium* may be harbored in animal spoors – how did that idea get transformed to needing tetanus shots after the slightest most antiseptic nick around the house?

Ask your doctor about the last case of tetanus he saw.

DPT CONTAMINANTS

Let's not forget that for 80 years DPT had been "stabilized" with thimerosal - a mercury compound - and also contains formaldehyde - a carcinogenic embalming fluid, (*PDR*) [75] Mercury causes nerve damage; formaldehyde causes cancer. Can't imagine why there would be so many

REACTIONS

Other reactions to DPT include the following: [229]

death	**vomiting**
permanent neurological damage	**convulsions**
high-pitched screaming	**anaphylactic shock**
encephalopathy [brain fever]	**muscle spasms**

Know any babies who start screaming soon after a shot? For decades there have been frequent references to the characteristic "high-pitched screaming" associated with DPT shots. One comment made by the authors of the UCLA study is highly expressive of the overall IQ often encountered in the field of "immunization":

"Unusual high-pitched screaming has been previously reported after DPT immunization. Several authors feel that this should be categorized as a major reaction; however, the significance of this reaction is unknown." *Pediatrics* [229]

Unknown? How about that the helpless little being who has just set foot on earth is in intense distress from the toxic assault on its unformed central nervous system and is frightened to death, not knowing if it will survive... how's that for a hypothesis? It's quite far-fetched and could only be verified by "controlled scientific study," of course... Till then, let's continue assaulting our defenseless children, disregarding their outcry.

There's no mystery about high-pitched screaming. Coulter (p 32) [227] has a whole section of cited medical studies dating from 1961 correlating the screaming and crying with irritation of the nervous system. It dovetails perfectly with later studies on mercury and autism. (Geier) [105]

How much education do you need to figure this out?

NEUROLOGICAL DAMAGE WITH DPT

Most of the adverse effects of DPT are symptoms of damage to the nervous system. It's no wonder - the concentrated pertussis bacteria is one of the most toxic compounds that exist. The result is a class of vaccine known as a **toxoid**, which simply means a "controlled" poison. Mercury continued to be used as a preservative in the DPT vaccine even though it has been known for decades that mercury poisoning causes brain damage by chemically attacking the nerve cells. (Widman, Bernard, Cave) [207, 180, 185]

Now consider the formative brain and nervous system in a two-month-old infant. Nerve connections are still being formed; nerve insulation (**myelin**) begins at birth. We all know that babies develop at different rates: some walk and talk sooner than others, etc. Same with the nervous system. No studies have ever been done to prove that at two months old, the nervous system has developed to a point where it is capable of withstanding an environment containing mercury and formaldehyde. That would be impossible, because of the wide variation in infant development. That's why most of Europe vaccinates at two years, to give the immune system at least a fighting chance at development. But by that time an American baby has already had **36 vaccines**!

Dozens of studies since 1933 (Madsen) [234] found significant numbers of nerve-damaged DPT babies, even with the systematic under-reporting cited above. The correlation has been made, yet we keep vaccinating. And now we're up to 5 separate shots of DPT, the only country in the world requiring that many.

DPT or DTaP?

By 1996, so many adverse reactions were being pinned on the *Pertussis* component that the marketing department realized it was time for a new and improved version. Enter the acellular pertussis vaccine. Hawked as the safer pertussis vaccine because it contained no whole bacterial cells, the acellular vaccine contains enough byproducts of the bacteria that it is supposedly still able to trigger the magical antibody response without causing all those nasty deaths and side effects we got from the old-fashioned DPT. Was any new long-term testing done in combination with DT before the vaccine was released? Three guesses.

Don't be taken in by the whole cell/acellular shell game. In terms of overall toxicity to a newborn infant's blood, the distinction is not worth making. The vaccine is still #1 for vaccine injury cases.

Ever wonder what happened to all those millions of doses of DPT stockpiled in storage when DTaP came out? Answer: nothing. Even though the dangers of DPT supposedly necessitated the development of the new DTaP, doctors are still entitled to use the old mercury-laced DPT vaccine all they want, because it's still a licensed product.

Or the surplus may just be dumped in Third World markets.

SIDS AND DPT

Australian researcher Viera Scheibner PhD stumbled onto the link between Sudden Infant Death syndrome and DPT by accident. Her husband had developed a breathing monitor for infants, to try and prevent SIDS.

The Scheibners noticed distinct patterns of distress after monitoring hundreds of babies. They discovered a 16-day crisis following DPT shots - the pattern was unmistakable. Then they correlated their findings with many other studies, including the 200 SIDS babies in Tennessee, and found the exact same pattern.

Scheibner's work has been vigorously suppressed in many places, like the USA for example. In Australia however, their unrelenting efforts put an end to mandatory DPT shots.   [239]

In 1983 there was a study done at the Los Angeles County Coroner's Office correlating DPT with SIDS. Researchers were intrigued by a recent CDC investigation of 200 Tennessee babies who died 24 hours after DPT shots, and wanted to see if there were any correlation. So the Los Angeles group interviewed parents of 145 recent SIDS victims. Here's what they found:

Of the 145 SIDS deaths, 53 had been recently DPT-immunized, at the following intervals:

> **51% had been given DPT within 4 weeks of death**
> **32% within 1 week of death**
> **11% within 1 day of death**

Researchers decided theses numbers were "statistically significant." (Baraff) [230] Very astute.

GLOBAL DPT

There have been many other formal studies correlating DPT with SIDS. [227] So many problems are seen with the DPT vaccine that few countries in the world still force it. Sweden halted it in 1979. (Trollfors) [231] Even though the incidence of whooping cough then increased slightly, the disease is much milder in form, and no Swedish babies have died from it since. And once somebody gets the disease, they have true natural, lifetime immunity. Which is more than we can say for DPT shots.

Similar sequences happened in Japan, West Germany, Britain, and other European countries. When they stopped vaccinating, the disease returned in a milder form, but babies aren't dying from it. The key is: **not one country started the vaccine up again** after discontinuing it. And the only country left in western Europe with compulsory pertussis vaccination is Iceland. ([227] p 95)

Other reactions from pertussis vaccine include: [244]

anaphylactic shock	**encephalopathy**
death	**brachial neuritis**
convulsions	**Guillain-Barre**
hives	**rash**
joint pain	**low blood pressure**
difficulty breathing	**swelling of the mouth**
infantile spasms	**bulging fontanelle**

These are the precise symptoms of acute mercury poisoning. (Bernard, [180])

ONCE BITTEN TWICE SHY

Since Toomey's article in the 1949 issue of *JAMA* [228], most medical journal articles about DPT agree on one thing: any child who has had a reaction should not be given the vaccine again in the future. Same for a child who has any family history of neuro-logical disorders or "illness of any kind." This recommendation is very consistent throughout the literature, and since 1975 has been the official stance of the World Health Organization. It is strictly followed in England, Sweden, and the Netherlands. (p129 [227]) Even the CDC's own morbidity reports (*MMWR* vol.36) state that children with a family history of convulsions are nine times more likely to have a seizure following a DPT shot. [232]

IGNORE THE EXPERTS

So it is imponderable that in actual practice in the U.S., there's just no room for such a simple screening procedure. Children are **never** screened by pediatricians to rule out those who are deemed high risk by the manufacturer itself. Apparently, it doesn't make political sense, and therefore almost no pediatrician would ever track reactions to DPT or reject a child simply because he has a history of central nervous system problems, or of prior reactions to the shot. Such a decision would single out that doctor as a troublemaker who was "making waves."

The arrogance of American doctors being able to ignore this worldwide dictum of medical procedure speaks volumes about the political controls mandating vaccination in this country, wouldn't you say? The American Association of Pediatricians has defied the unified medical opinion of the rest of the world with statements like: "A family history of convulsions or neurological disorders is not a contraindication." (*APA Red Book*) [246]   Pretty cheeky, even for them.

DPT: THE ONE TO SKIP

If you could choose one shot in the whole arsenal to skip, DPT would be the one. Fully **75% of the $2 billion** in vaccine damages paid out by VICP since 1991 has been awarded for reactions from DPT. (Goodwin, Dodd [179, 314, 35])

DOES THE DPT VACCINE REALLY WORK?

Even with a 77% DPT vaccination rate in the U.S. there are still 17,000 cases of pertussis per year, mostly in California.

"In 2010, 9,477 cases of pertussis (including ten infant deaths) were reported throughout California. This is the most cases reported in 65 years.."   [123]

And the number has been rising steadily since 1980. (CDC [123]) Reason: the "immunity" wears off in a few years. This leaves the individual open to the disease later in life, in an **atypical form**, which is more serious. Then the adults with the atypical form may expose it to infants who are totally unprotected from this new disease.

It is the vaccine creating the atypical form.

The other problem is that increasing numbers of unvaccinated infants are now being exposed to these brand new atypical forms of pertussis. It will take generations to develop species immunity to the new atypical forms.

A 1994 article in the *NEJM* showed that 80% of children under 5 who got pertussis had been fully vaccinated. The researchers concluded that the vaccine offered insufficient protection from the disease. [300]

There have been several local outbreaks of a few hundred cases of pertussis in the past 6 years, in Colorado, Oregon, New Mexico, California and other states. Obviously all these DPT shots have not had their advertised effect over the years. Since 2005, there are 5 doses in the Mandated Schedule for US children. [55] In outbreak situations, the response by local health authorities has usually been to add yet another dose - #6 - of this most toxic of vaccines to the already overloaded infant immune system, even though about 90% of the sick children in these locales have already been vaccinated with multiple doses of DPT.

So here's the picture: not only are children exposed to many possible side effects, but the actual promised benefit itself - immunity - never gets delivered. More, more, and more doses of the same vaccine cannot help. First they said 3 doses were enough, then 4, then 5, then 6. And now 5 more for adults. Medspeak has twisted the concept of immunity. True immunity is for life. It does not come in a syringe.

New research from the very credible Age of Autism site has a peer-reviewed study from the *International Journal of Epidemiology*, flatly demonstrating the raw mortality data among African children from a single dose of DPT vaccine. [22] **Deaths doubled after a single dose, quadrupled after a second and third dose**. This corroborates with US VICP mortality statistics showing the **DPT is the single most dangerous shot ever created, "harming more children than saving."** [5]

THE QUESTION

Is it really worth the risk to expose two-month-old infants to a toxin with all the above side effects in order to provide an imaginary temporary "immunity" which wears off a few months later, requiring a booster shot? And all this for a disease that was disappearing anyway?

Only the tip of the pertussis vaccine iceberg is presented here; there's so much data, most of it from mainstream medical sources. It's far worse than this section suggests. The reader is directed to the sources cited for a more in-depth look.

SHAKEN BABY SYNDROME

The 1990s brought a new phenomenon: a disease created by media and district attorneys. Suddenly, they told us, people have started killing their own babies by shaking them to death, in mass numbers. For spin value, they came up with a name: **Shaken Baby Syndrome.**

Many experts, like John Menkes, MD of Cedars Sinai, said at the outset that Shaken Baby Syndrome was often a vehicle for a local DA to get his name in the paper, while in reality the fatal side effects of DPT were being covered up. (Goodwin) [179]   [106]

A leading expert on SBS is certainly San Diego attorney Toni Blake. [312] Some astounding figures appear on her website SBSdefense.com:

- 1500 SBS cases per year
- about a 75% conviction rate once charged
- once in prison, less than 5% are ever freed

The neurological picture of the SBS baby can be identical to reactions from the DPT vaccine. The signs are

intracranial hemorrhage
cerebral edema
subdural hematoma.

These 3 symptoms became the famous **triad** widely used by the legal players who have reaped the greatest personal benefit in crafting this imaginary new crimewave.

'Expert' witnesses, some charging $10,000 per day, [95] now derive enormous fortunes traveling from town to town, offering their opinions for hire to apply to any and all defendants unlucky enough to have been in the proximity of an infant who collapses with one of these triad symptoms, whatever the actual cause. ([95], note 174)

In this strange new criminal arena, many cases have been convicted just by demonstrating even one of the triad, orchestrated by DAs with unlimited coffers for expert witnesses, and judges who guide juries to an opinion. If all 3 triad findings are present, the term **pathognomonic** was floated: for several years the hired guns have convinced juries the presence of the infallible triad absolutely proved that the baby had to have been intentionally shaken to death by the nearest human. With no witnesses, no other evidence. Thousands are in jail on that Inquisitorial decision.

In recent years, newer science has shown that the 'triad' no longer definitively proves SBS. ([95, note 110)   Many other events can cause the same exact neuronal damage:

- **normal birth   [82]**
- **previous injury**
- **short distance fall**
- **non-traumatic injury**
- **pre-existing subdural hematoma [312]**

A study in the journal *Radiology* [82] has discovered that **26% of normal births** result in **intracranial hemorrhage**, detectable on MRI, but which never cause any apparent symptoms. It has been known for years in the SBS defense community that at least **75%** of SBS cases already have records of old subdural hematomas by the date of the arrest. [312]

Unfortunately, the SBS industry has become so well funded, with such a foundation of legal decisions, such a juggernaut of social and economic pressure that the new science has not been readily accepted into the body of "law."   They just haven't kept up. Convictions are still coming down today based solely on obsolete triad symptoms, out of date science. If focused primarily on self aggrandizement, the new industry would see little benefit in keeping current on the true science of neurological injury.

SCIENCE IS NOT WHATEVER THE EXPERTS SAY

The fundamental error that prosecutors have successfully sold is that science is whatever comes out of the mouth of the paid experts. But that's not necessarily science. Real science is the first to admit its own limitations and margins of error. It is broad by definition. True scientific method always acknowledges that our understanding in every field of inquiry is in flux, is always adding to its own refinement with each new study, and is always asking the next question.

This is the opposite of what the DAs, judges and 'expert' witnesses in the SBS industry often pawn off as science. They seem to have carved out their tiny little area of neurological research, have locked it off, frozen it in time, and guard it ferociously, with all the formidable resources they now command. They pretend that the subject is closed, not open to further inquiry, and now they know everything that can possibly be known about this type of traumatic brain injury. In a masterpiece of self promotion, these skilled actors continue to convince juries that the triad of symptoms can absolutely override any and all other circumstances of a case. Thus may a trial be open to the flagrant prostitution and abuse of a very small, isolated corner of research, now unassailable and permanent, the very antithesis of science.   [106]

MILLION$ TO FEED NEW INDUSTRY

In the broad strokes, the Shaken Baby mythology has now hit the motherlode – colossal funding [49] for 'research' that proves its own myopic theories, fosters its own growth, and provides a deep trough to feed all players – researchers, 'expert' witnesses, anyone who can add to the monolith of biased evidence to keep the show rolling along. If that can only happen by destroying the lives of a steady supply of hapless defendants who were in the wrong place at the wrong time, so be it.

Shocking that the children's hospitals have become prime participants in this dark game. With the funding they receive from the top, they train their staff to be fiercely vigilant for any case that can be made to fit the mold: arrest, prosecution, and conviction. Today the #**1 risk factor** in being charged with SBS is if the child is taken first to a children's hospital. This means if your child has a true accidental head injury, if you want to avoid being falsely accused of SBS, the last place on earth you want to go is a children's hospital. [312] [106]

Remember, we are not talking about child abuse here. No punishment is sufficient for actual perpetrators of those particular crimes. Rather, we're talking about set-ups – the systematic framing of innocent people in order to feed a bloated new industry.

NOW FOR THE BAD NEWS

In reviewing the legal literature of SBS cases [95] one fact stands out with glaring intensity: **vaccine injury** has been systematically eliminated from the entire discussion. Despite more than $2 billion paid out in vaccine injuries, million dollar settlements for diagnoses like PDD – Pervasive Developmental Disorder, etc, the prodigious amount of research documenting neurological damage and death from mercury, aluminum, MMR vaccines, and DPT vaccines cited in this book, the possibility of classic triad symptoms resulting from vaccines has simply been banished from legal literature on SBS.   Defense attorneys don't even bring it up.

Taking all the medical documentation of brain injury from vaccines, as listed in the Reference section below, and with the number of childhood vaccines having tripled since the 1980s, it is likely that the vast majority of cases labeled Shaken Baby Syndrome have been caused by vaccine injury. More than likely.

MEASLES

Measles is a mild, self-limiting, immune-building viral disease of childhood. Symptoms are red spots on the skin and mouth, fever, and fatigue. Commonly resolves in a week.

Most of those who grew up in the 1950s remember getting measles. Not a big deal. And they got lifetime immunity in the bargain. Natural immunity. (*Merck*, p 1098) [266]

Looking at the Figure 2 above, we see the disease almost completely disappeared by itself before mass vaccinations became popular in the late 1960s.

Measles vaccine was part of the MMR (measles-mumps-rubella) vaccine package developed in the early 1970s. Once again, it wouldn't be so bad if the vaccine were simply unnecessary. But an entire array of side effects can result from the MMR vaccine:

loss of muscle control	**meningitis**	**seizures**
mental retardation	**Reye's Syndrome**	**diabetes**
paralysis	**anaphylactic shock**	**MS**
Guillain-Barre Syndrome	**bloodclot**	**encephalitis**

But the reason the MMR vaccine was sold to the public in the first place was to protect against **encephalitis**. Now here it's listed as a side effect of the vaccine? Measles itself doesn't cause all these illnesses. Even pediatricians know that the vaccine contains a "slow virus" that can hide in tissues for years, and then manifest later in life. This is why so many doctors in Los Angeles refused to use the MMR vaccine on their own children. (Mendelsohn, p 237,238) [241]

A 1996 report stated that the measles vaccine

"produces immune suppression which contributes to an increased susceptibility to other infections."
     - *Clinical Immunology and Pathology*, [Auwerter, 197]

Let me get this right. Not only does the measles vaccine not prevent measles; it also increases the chances of getting other infections?

Looks like the vaccine's worse than the disease. And we have mandated such a vaccine for the general population based on undocumented claims of possible encephalitis?

With measles specifically, the **absence of antibodies** after vaccination has been known for decades:

"Antibody production is therefore not necessary either for recovery from or for the development of immunity to measles." - Nobel laureate, Sir MacFarlane Burnet, 1971 [201]

Let's trace the vaccine's **effectiveness** for preventing measles. By 1978, half the cases of measles were found in vaccinated children.

And the WHO stated that those vaccinated have a 15 times greater chance of catching measles than those not vaccinated! ([241], p 238)

Between 1983 and 1989, incidence of measles **increased 10-fold**. In the next year, incidence increased another 50 percent! 1990 saw 27,000 cases and 100 deaths reported in the U.S. (p 511) [263]

Furthermore the CDC itself reports measles outbreaks in

populations with 100% vaccination rates! Their "explanation": "...the apparent paradox is that **measles...becomes a disease of immunized persons.**" (*MMWR*, Oct 1984) [286]

What about the value of childhood measles as an immune-building experience? Viera Scheibner: [247]

"It is well known that measles is an **important milestone in the maturing process of children.** Why would anybody want to delay the maturation process of children and their immune systems?"

The real horror about the measles vaccine, however, didn't explode into public awareness till the House of Representatives hearings on autism, convened by Dan Burton on 6 April 2000. Research done in England and Ireland began to show the measles vaccine as one of the two most likely causes of autism.

HEMOPHILUS INFLUENZAE TYPE B MENINGITIS

Today a "meningitis vaccine" (HiB) is routinely given to infants at 2, 4, 6, and 12 months of age.

This disease has nothing to do with influenza or flu shots. Confusing *H. influenzae* with flu is a common error, even among pediatricians. In fact, that's a good screening question.

Hemophilus influenzae bacteria were originally so named because they were thought to be found in people who had the flu. Later, researchers discovered that the bacteria are found in mucous membranes of normal people, but the name stuck.

H. influenzae may occur with many mild self-limiting infections of a child's nose and throat. (Neustadter, p.161) [215] On very rare occasions, a certain strain of *H. influenzae* (Type B) can also be seen with meningitis, usually in children. The incidence has actually been increasing since the 1960s, as has the number of vaccines given to children. The solution? Another vaccine!

Early HiB vaccine research took place in Finland. In a study of **100,000 subjects**, HiB was found to have **no efficacy at all** under 18 months of age. (Peltola *Pediatrics* vol. 60, 1977) [242] by which age American children have already had **three separate shots**! Below 24 months, the vaccine was "uncertain."

In 1986, the *New England Journal of Medicine* published a follow-up study of 55 cases of HiB disease, all of whom had been vaccinated. 39 got meningitis, and 3 died. Six others went deaf. (Granoff) [243]

In a massive study in Norway in 1988 of over **171,000 subjects**, the vaccine's "effect was insufficient to justify a public vaccination programme." (Bjune) [285] The incidence of HiB meningitis dropped from 300 cases per year in 1988 to 200 cases in 1991 on its own, without mandatory vaccination.

The first of the HiB vaccines, which was called **PRP**, didn't work very well. In the usual tradition of testing a vaccine on the live population, by 1988 PRP was actually causing more cases of the disease than it was preventing. (*JAMA* [291]) The way this happened was that the child would contract a mild version of *H. influenzae* in the nose or throat, which normally would have self-resolved. But because the child had been vaccinated, the immune system was suppressed, thereby allowing the disease to penetrate deeper into the nervous system, and to set up shop in the meninges (lining of the spinal cord). After thousands of children were experimentally inoculated, PRP was eventually abandoned.

A well-documented side effect of HiB vaccination is a marked increase in **infant diabetes**. Here are three studies. Bolded year denotes start of HiB vaccination.

Location	year	infant diabetes/100,000
Finland	1966-75	12
	1981	16
	1984	19
	1988	26
	1991	29

source: *Inf Dis in Clin Pract* vol 6 1997 p.449

Pittsburgh	1975-84	6
	1985-94	13

source: *Diabetes Care* vol 21 1998 p. 1278   [288]

England	1992-93	14
	1994	22

- *Brit Med J* 1997 p.713 [287]

We're talking about diabetes in infants, less than 4 years old! Before the 1960s, such a phenomenon was unknown. Vaccines doubled between 1960 and 1980.

Hemophilus influenzae vaccine (HiB) contained aluminum and mercury, toxins whose effects we have seen above.

Like all vaccines, *H. influenzae* is always being tested - on your children. No one noticed how they dropped down from four doses to three on the Schedule starting in 2006, for no reason. Then in

2007, back up to 4.   Politics, not science.

INFLUENZA AND INFLUENZA SHOTS

No relation to *H. influenzae* vaccine, flu vaccines are a fairly recent development, and also very big business.

A little research in the area of influenza vaccine reveals a wasteland of disinformation and political maneuvering.

Influenza is a virus that has the ability to be constantly reinventing itself throughout the population during a single season. The vaccine supposedly contains some versions of the causative agents, in a weakened form. With influenza, by the time the virus is isolated, cultured for manufacture, and distributed to the population, the current strain of virus has usually changed to a form completely unaffected by the vaccine! Michael Decker MD of Aventis, the flu vaccine manufacturer, laments: "By the time you know what's the right strain, you can't do anything about it." [116]

Penetrating observation.

The sicker the individual, or the greater the number of people with the virus, the faster it mutates. Scientists refer to such a trend as **gene amplification**. (Garrett, pp 578, 580, 614) [223]

This doesn't even take into account the unique form influenza virus takes within each person, or each city. Yet with flu shots, it's One Size Fits All - everyone gets the same vaccine. If it really worked, you wouldn't have to come back next year. Real immunity is for life.

SUCCESS FOR FLU VACCINE

On 7 Feb 05, after 20 years of lobbying, influenza finally made it onto the Schedule. The flu shot was quietly moved from the High Risk category to the regular Mandated Schedule. Suddenly it was recommended at 6 months and yearly thereafter until age 18. That raised the total number of mandated vaccines for an American child from **40 to 58** in one fell swoop.

No media covered the event.

WHY FLU SHOTS DON'T WORK

There are literally hundreds of strains of influenza virus present at any given time across the US. During any flu season, the virus mutates several times, not only in any given locale, but even within individuals. This simple fact explains why the flu vaccine has never been effective at reducing either deaths or incidence of influenza in this country during the past 20 years.

Ever notice that people who get flu shots all the time keep getting the flu? Could that have anything to do with not giving the body a chance to put immunity together for itself?

One problem might be that flu vaccine has always contained **mercury**. (*PDR*, 2010) And also **formaldehyde and ethylene glycol**. [244]

With such a composition, it is not surprising that the flu vaccine doesn't prevent the flu. Even the CDC only claims a **44% 'success rate'** for flu vaccine. [65]   In truth, it's much lower.   Taking a closer look at the 'research' from which CDC is making its claims, it begins to dawn on you that there are no real clinical trials, no actual risk-to-benefit studies: the 'testing' is done by giving the best-guess vaccine to the live population and then following up with unfounded editorializing from epidemiological data.

Echoing the same sentiments towards flu shots, England's top medical publication *British Medical Journal* found that when it comes to influenza vaccine,   [108]

"Evidence from systematic reviews shows that inactivated **vaccines have little or no effect**... Most **studies are of poor methodological quality** and the impact of confounders is high. **Little comparative evidence exists on the safety of these vaccines**."

Such de-evolution of scientific policy makes perfect sense, considering the way flu vaccines are funded and manufactured. In Oct 2008, one of the world's largest flu vax companies, the Belgian conglomerate Solvay Pharmaceuticals, cancelled their plans to build a new flu vaccine plant in Marietta GA, even though they were getting 60% of construction costs from the US government to build the plant, and even though they had already received $300 million two years earlier to develop flu vaccines! [66] Solvay's reason for backing out: the flu vaccine market is '**uncertain and weakening.**' They're referring to the declining confidence of people in flu shots, as more and more people are seeing the vaccinated come down with the flu:

Unsold doses of flu vaccine

2006   18 million of 121 million doses
2007   27 million of 140 million doses   [66]

Such figures did not bode well for venture capital. Solvay is a business - this isn't about health or the well being of the American people or any such happy nonsense as that. There are only 5 companies in the world who make flu vaccine; Solvay makes only flu vaccine. It can't be taking the same risks as the recipients of its vaccine...

This was the dejected economic climate in the flu vax business when swine flu popped up out of nowhere in 2009. All at once, it was nothing but blue sky...

FLU SHOTS AND ALZHEIMERS

Does it seem like Alzheimer's was getting more common the past

decade? Hugh Fudenburg, MD a leading immunogeneticist, with some 850 papers peer-reviewed, told us why back in 2000:

"If an individual had 5 consecutive flu shots between 1970 and 1980, the chances of Alzheimer's Disease was 10 times greater than for those getting... no shots."   [298]

Think that might have anything to do with the aluminum?

The new Adult Schedule recommends yearly shots until 60. [26]

ADULT SHOTS AND HOOKS

Panic among the vaccine sales force may help to explain the magical appearance of the Adult Immunization Schedule suddenly in early 2008 in which every adult was now to be scheduled for **45 flu shots after the age of 18!** [26] Ad mavens have successfully targeted the elderly, who now get 72% of all flu shots even though they are most susceptible to the aluminum. [66]

A standard hook now in vaccine marketing repertoire is 'pandemic,' starting with the nonexistent Avian flu of 2005. As that chimera faded off into the boneyard of plague hysteria memorabilia, [52] the sales team next scored a sterling success with the 2009 swine flu 'outbreak.' Venture capital prospects were never brighter.

SWINE FLU: BOUTIQUE PANDEMIC OF 2009

The first and most important rule in creating any epidemic is that the marketing of the disease cannot outpace the rate of the disease itself. When doom and gloom predictions are too overstated, the entire purpose of the whole program is defeated –which was, selling the vaccine. Getting people to show up for it.

The 2009 swine flu/H1N1 disaster made that fatal error, hiring the best publicists money can buy. The scenario they painted was so grim, the threat so dire that no set of actual events short of the Bubonic Plague could have lived up to it. So we witnessed the unravelling of a 'pandemic' before enough people showed up to participate in it. Even the impaired mentality of the general public saw through that veil. After all those months of threats and hysteria from every level of government, in all media, the American people said no thanks, we're not buying swine flu.

A complete summary of the 2009 H1N1 sideshow may be found online in the chapters *Swine Flu: Global Pandemic* and *Goodbye Swine Flu* [48] So much bad science and self-serving propaganda was dumped onto the public regarding this cheap promotion that it would fill this book, but the important lesson we must take from it is to apprehend the pattern of the made-to-order pandemic that has now become firmly entrenched in our culture, and can be trotted out on command. **The Boutique Epidemic**.

Here are just a few details from those chapters on the 2009 Swine Flu fiasco, to keep us mindful of standard techniques of persuasion and misdirection we can expect from now on in marketing new vaccines.

SWINE FLU APRIL 2009

The original Swine Flu Vaccine program of **1976** was the worst vaccine disaster in US history, with some **21 deaths** and almost **600** people paralyzed [48] Eventually the government paid out almost **$400 million** in claims - for a disease that never existed. [48]

With a history like that, it is astounding that policymakers would want to use that same label again. The next mention of swine flu was not until 30 years later, in April 2009. It began with conflicting reports of several hundred Mexicans 'infected' with swine flu, 150 of whom were 'believed to have' died from it.

In the first 4 days, the word **pandemic** was already present in all media stories - a tip-off for the massive promo about to be unleashed.

The hysteria gathered momentum as government officials fell over each other to make the most dire predictions possible.

IGNITING THE HYSTERIA

Americans got a valuable lesson from the rabid way the government spokesmen kindled the fire those first weeks. Rather than report simply that there was a possible new illness and that it's under investigation, everyone immediately rang the Doomsday Bell. With no solid data, W.H.O.'s Margaret Chan irresponsibly declared "a public health emergency of international concern." (WHO Health Advisory, April 2009, [58])

Chan followed that up with the unfounded 11 June declaration of a Phase 6 "Pandemic Emergency." Media had a bloodfest over that announcement. [59]

Chan's next hysterical outburst came on 16 July 09:

"modeling suggests that swine flu has an **attack rate of 30%** — once it enters a country, the likelihood is 30% of citizens will catch it at some point...."

Modeling? Is that like channeling? Obviously a vaccine was being promoted here. But it was her next phrase that hung the WHO out to dry:

"One should be available soon, in August. But having a vaccine available is not the same as having a vaccine that is proven safe. Clinical trial data will not be available for another two to three months." [57]

Chan knew she was at sea here. New vaccines take at least a year to develop. As we have seen, swine flu vaccine clinical trials only began in August 2009. So it was astounding when five weeks later the FDA approved an H1N1 vaccine!   [47]

WHAT IS WHO?

For the 2009 H1N1 show, WHO's prime source of information was a committee calling itself the European Scientific Working Group on Influenza, who it turns out is funded entirely by the 5 manufacturers who ended up with the H1N1 vaccine contracts. JP Morgan estimated that as a result of that one WHO declaration of pandemic, the vax makers stood to gain up to **$15 billion**. [60]

What we're seeing by 2009 was the **privatization of WHO**. Along with its collaborators, WHO had built a machine around the impending pandemic. [61] No problem when H1N1 fizzles; we now have the technology to whip up another Boutique Epidemic at any time. With five false epidemics in the past eight years, the pattern is now well tested. And that was the prime lesson we must take from swine flu 2009.

H1N1: CREATING THE VILLAIN

For the first 2 months, H1N1 was not even mentioned. The cases were just called swine flu - some weird new strain of pig virus. It was only when the bacon industry kept complaining to Obama that the H1N1 characterization was hit upon. [51], Kugler]

The first cases of swine flu were coming from Third World areas where even basic medical services are lacking, let alone a sophisticated screening test for a brand new disease. That procedure would take months to create, even in the most modern of clinical settings.

So once again we ask, without a screening procedure, exactly what were they counting, in Mexico, in Texas, wherever? What set these cases apart from ordinary flu?

WHAT A TANGLED WEB WE WEAVE

CDC's brilliant solution was H1N1, even though they knew that made no sense either, with over 700 strains. But they had to call it something, so by June 2009 the CDC's official title for the new pandemic was the **2009 H1N1 Influenza A.** [55]

Ludicrously apparent to anyone who was eventually going to put the pieces of the puzzle together, suddenly switching names and calling the new disease H1N1 flu was a patent attempt to lump any Class A flu into the H1N1 category.

Equally embarrassing was the CDC statement of 3 Oct 09 in which they printed the utterly insupportable pronouncement that "a total of **99% of circulating influenza viruses in the United States were 2009 H1N1 influenza**."   ([40] Barclay)

THE SWINE FLU PROGRAM UNRAVELS

The first death knell for the 2009 vaccine hoax was sounded on 21 Sep 09 in an article that appeared in *Associated Press*. [43] The article stated that the first of the swine flu vaccines were to come out in October.

National Institutes of Health was recommending four separate flu shots to kids younger than 10 years old. Two of the shots would be the brand new untested swine flu vaccines, and the other two the 'regular' flu shot.

NIH director Tony Fauci and CDC's Ann Schuchat proclaimed:

- children 9 and under will need 2 flu shots and 2 swine flu shots
- everybody else will need 1 of each
- 251 million doses will be ready in October
- kids can get both shots the same day, one in each arm
- NIH has studies involving 600 children
- children 10 and older showed protection from the new vaccine
- a second dose is necessary to 'rev up' the immune system

CDC's Schuchat, towering medical genius, obviously off her meds that day, then piped in "it will be OK for kids to get one shot in each arm on the same visit." Excuse us, Dr Mengele? Did you remember in first quarter pre-med when you learned that both arms were attached to the same body? Exactly what clinical trials confirm this personal hallucination of yours?

In every declining civilization in history, this has been a hallmark of unanchored officials: making unchallenged idiotic statements.

THE FORMATIVE INFANT IMMUNE SYSTEM

One final comment from NIH's Tony Fauci:

"Younger children simply "don't have as mature an immune system," Fauci explained. "So a first dose of vaccine against a flu strain they've never experienced acts as an introduction for their immune system, and a booster shortly thereafter revs up that immune response " [46]

Wow. Let's take a breath here. For the first time in history we had the director of the National Institutes of Health enunciating in a worldwide forum one of the principal reasons why young children might not be vaccinated at all: **they don't have a mature immune system.** Absolutely true. No child is born with an intact immune system. That very complex biological symphony of interrelated allergic responses, antibodies, antigens, self recognition, cell response, etc -- about which we still have only the vaguest knowledge -- struggles its way into existence during the early years of the child's life. It needs no help, no interference, no enormous experimental toxic load, especially one so politically contrived, in its fight to survive.

SWINE FLU VACCINE CLINICAL TRIALS

In one of the five swine flu vaccine clinical trials, the one by Sanofi Pasteur [47] we learn that their trial began in August 2009 and would go until April 2010. The sample size was 650 children. The shocking fact in the article is that Sanofi stated that the after **5 weeks** of testing, the FDA had just approved their H1N1 vaccine!

Traditionally it takes at least a year to develop and test a new vaccine. Five weeks was a new world record.

SEPT. SURPRISE: UNRESTRICTED MERCURY IN NEW VAX

On 29 Sept 09, another shocker arrived: the new swine flu vaccines may contain unlimited levels of mercury! Washington State Health Secretary Salecky announced [42] that the state of Washington just lifted allowable limits of thimerosal in the new swine flu vaccines, with no new levels set.

The announcement was masterfully phrased, obviously the work of professional publicists:

"**Lifting mercury limits** for H1N1 vaccine will give pregnant women and parents or guardians of children under three the option of getting the vaccine if they want it."

Couching the issue in terms of availability to pregnant women sidesteps the obvious: it would also give these women the option of exposing themselves and their unborn children to unrestricted levels of the third most lethal neurotoxin known to man: organic mercury, not to mention manmade viral mutations.

The Washington State declaration quoted Sanofi Pasteur - from its 15 Sep 09 announcement [47] that their new swine flu vaccination had just been licensed by the FDA.

The spectre of thimerosal having been raised portends that the manufacturers who have just been awarded these huge contracts to rush a vaccine onto the market -- that the new vaccines may not be new at all, but rather old stockpiled vaccines that have been sitting around for years: either old flu vaccines or Avian flu vaccines, or virtually anything with a fragment of any flu virus. What else could they be, after just 5 weeks?

H1N1 VACCINE MISCARRIAGES

The urgency over the 2009 swine flu program was being stoked almost daily by inflammatory news stories, all with the same slant: no time to test these new vaccines. So let's just get them out there to the children and pregnant women such as they are. We'll sort out the details later.

Details like toxicity, lethal side effects, permanent neurological damage, autism, genome alteration, etc.

CDC Director Thomas Frieden on 60 Minutes:

"We're confident it will be effective, and we have every reason to believe that it will be safe." [62]

Empty words. Without complete clinical trials, nothing is really known about either the safety or the efficacy of any vaccine. From a national health perspective, we have taken a dodgey turn indeed if we can replace standard protocols for testing and licensing vaccines with hollow statements from regulatory officials, implying clinical testing is no longer necessary. If the substances being thus green-lighted had no side effects, that would be one thing. Quite another here, in light of the limitless amounts of allowable mercury, as well as the other potential effects of an untested vaccine being not only licensed for use, but also most aggressively marketed and promoted for the general public, especially children and pregnant women.

A few Americans did fall for the ruse however and got vaccinated. Reported reactions were met with routine denials. But some effects were too obvious to deny. Like the 10 Sep 2011 headline about the thousands of US women miscarrying after the H1N1 vaccine. [2] Again, a story that was largely buried.

One fact is certain: without hyperbole or sensationalism, the new swine flu vaccine - unidentified, untested and untried - would have been the most dangerous immunological experiment on this country's children in history. If the people would have bought it.

GOODBYE SWINE FLU

What happened to SARS? Where is it? What happened to anthrax, smallpox, Avian flu, mad cow— they're gone. And they won't be back. They served their purpose – terrorize and distract – spend billions for new pharmaceuticals, unproven and ultimately unnecessary. Afterwards the threats always vanish, like the dew off the new grass in the morning sun — gone. [48]

Despite last-ditch attempts to salvage sales of unwanted vaccines, by early 2010 the swine flu 'pandemic' had all but disappeared, behind some fast back-pedaling:

"with the second wave of H1N1 infections having crested in the United States, leading epidemiologists are predicting that the pandemic could end up ranking as the mildest since modern medicine began documenting influenza outbreaks" (Stein [62])

As demand fell, many states as well as most of the EU countries returned stocks of unused H1N1 vaccine. [24, 28] In Feb. and Mar. 2010, desperate attempts were made to try and salvage the sinking H1N1 ship, by proclaiming the 'pandemic' was still a threat and could re-emerge anywhere, etc.

Desperate to move dead stockpiles of a vaccine nobody wanted, in Feb 2010 they decided to include the unpopular H1N1 vaccine into the next year's regular flu shot. [27]

EUROPEAN INVESTIGATION OF FALSE PANDEMIC

By January 2010 the EU was mounting a full scale investigation of what they called "the false pandemic" engineered by the WHO in league with vaccine makers. [25, 30, 28] One investigative body – the **Parliamentary Assembly of the Council of Europe**, representing 47 countries, called the swine flu campaign of 2009 "one of the greatest medical scandals of the century."

Chaired by Germany's Wolfgang Wodarg, MD, PACE saw how the 2009 swine flu pandemic was created by **artificial re-categorization of normal flu** cases, and then marketed into an illusory global pandemic.

PACE members wondered about the intensity of the original dire pronouncements of WHO and CDC, , finding "no reason to sound the alarm at this level." This group of doctors and scientists then set out to track down the precise nature of the collusion between politicians and the drugmakers who received "sealed contracts" for vaccine production, before any legitimate science had validated an actual biological threat. Price tag for the new pandemic: **$18 billion**. [33]

Dr Wodarg discovered that in May 2010 the WHO had suddenly **changed its definition of pandemic**. The previous definition was that a pandemic had to be spreading in several countries, and had to be a very serious threat with an unusual number of proven deaths. Suddenly the new revised definition left out those requirements. The new pandemic had only to be a disease, not necessarily serious or deadly, that **seemed to be spreading** – within any country. [32, 33]

By late 2010 many countries had banned the H1N1 vaccine. Australia, Germany, Finland, and Switzerland to name a few.

In Sept 2010 Australians learned that their children were much more likely to end up in the hospital from the H1N1 vaccine than from the disease. [3]

LAST CALL FOR SWINE FLU

In stark contrast to the shrieking emergency headlines we had to endure for 2 years about H1N1 pandemic, suddenly all media was mute on the subject as though it never happened. When the American public rejected the vaccine, the states began to return their allotted stocks of vaccine. And then something unprecedented occurred: **the returned stockpiles were burned!** As though they were destroying evidence. [328] That has never happened in vaccine history.

After two losing forays into global vaccines, it is doubtful that swine flu will be back for some time. The vaccine was a failure and an embarrassment, and exposed the agenda and credibility of the regulating health agencies, for anyone who cared to put the pieces together.

But again we must ask: once the vaccine vanished from the scene, what happened to the threat of HIN1 flu? It's gone too. And not because the vaccine cured it, because people didn't get the vaccine. This flu is gone because it never existed in the first place.

THE RISE OF THE BOUTIQUE EPIDEMIC

Remember SARS? In Feb of 2003 suddenly a new infectious disease appeared in China, cause unknown. Worldwide panic ensued, quarantines, tourist economies devastated in Vietnam, Hong Kong, Canada, etc.

After inciting worldwide panic for almost 3 years, SARS was never proven to exist. No causative agent was ever identified. Looking at the WHO website during that time was just like watching H1N1 scores in 2009 - how many infected, how many deaths today, etc.

SARS eventually faded out as though it never happened. For a more complete history of its rise and fall: www.gulfwarvets.com

For those few keeping track, the SARS event offered a valuable lesson for the future. It followed the same contrived sequence that ushered in anthrax, smallpox, Avian flu, mad cow, swine flu:

• Claim a disease threat from a new bug
• Instill worldwide panic with unrelenting media
• Only hope of salvation: drugs and vaccines
• Spend the money
• Watch the threat vaporize

What happened to these global threats? They're gone. And they won't be back.

They served their purpose—terrorize and distract – and spend billions for new research, new pharmaceuticals, unproven and ultimately unnecessary.

The only value in remembering SARS is in discerning this pattern that is played out over and over. With world media anxiously waiting to pimp the next phony threat, perhaps the alert student could learn to be a little bit discriminating about what we can expect from the popular press, and to consider the underlying motivators for the sale of any new drugs or vaccines which will now mercifully save us all from the newest dire threat *du jour*.

Today the Boutique Epidemic is firmly engrained into our culture. Windfall profits of this magnitude are too great to resist when they can be garnered simply by following the same recipe for success demonstrated in the past 5 nonexistent diseases. It's a safe bet the next faux pandemic will be coming along before very long. It's just business. [32]

HEPATITIS A

After years of maneuvering, GlaxoSmithKline finally got their new vaccine for Hepatitis A tacked onto the mandated schedule in Jan 2002, with no public fanfare. [181]   The vaccine was called **Havrix**, and is delineated on p. 1456 of the 2007 *PDR*. [244]

WHAT IS HEPATITIS A?

Hepatitis A is an acute viral disease of the liver. Hepatitis A virus (HAV) has supposedly been isolated. [268]

How serious is this disease? Hepatitis A is a **mild, self limiting** disease, resolving on its own with no treatment in **4-8 weeks**. Most infections are **subclinical**, meaning that the people who get the disease never even know it because they never manifest symptoms. (Merck p 377) [266]

Most hepatitis A doesn't require treatment. Even the National Institutes of Health states that:

"Most people who have Hepatitis A get well on their own after a few weeks." [267] *NIH Manual*

Almost all cases of hepatitis A are found in Third World areas. So then why are we the only country in the world who recommends the vaccine on a mass scale, now forcing 4 doses on our children?

SYMPTOMS OF HEPATITIS A

According to the *Merck Manual* (p 382 [266]) the chief symptoms of hepatitis A are:

loss of appetite   NVD   hives   joint pain   dark urine

Hardly life-threatening situations. By the time these symptoms appear, the disease is no longer infectious.

Unlike hepatitis B, Type A hepatitis disappears completely after acute infection, and **does not contribute to chronic liver disease** or to cirrhosis. After the patient recovers, he has lifetime immunity. True immunity.

Hepatitis A is a disease of poor personal hygiene, bad sanitation, poverty, overcrowding - Third World scenario. Hepatitis A is not common in the United States.

OTHER CAUSES

It's shocking to discover that hepatitis can be caused by both hepatitis B and hepatitis C vaccines! This fact is found in a disclaimer that GlaxoSmithKlein makes about Havrix, that it can't cure the hepatitis caused by these other 2 vaccines. So can we infer from this that Havrix itself also causes hepatitis? We don't need to infer it. The manufacturer states it on p 1458 of the 2007 *PDR*: **a possible side effect of Havrix is hepatitis!** [244]

SO THEN WHAT'S THE VACCINE FOR?

The question arises - did we really need another vaccine beyond those already mandated for schoolkids, for a rare disease that resolves by itself in a few weeks?

Were there any studies done which prove that the new vaccine is safe when Havrix is added to the other mandated vaccines? No, there are none. The concept of **cumulative viral load** and its effect on the newborn is discussed above. Always disregarded.

HOW MANY CASES REALLY ARE THERE?

Finding the true incidence of the Hepatitis A in the US is a daunting task indeed. A standard government reference for epidemiology is *Statistical Abstracts*. On p 137 of the 2000 edition, we find that the overall incidence of Hepatitis A had been declining for the past two decades:

    1980 --- 29.1 cases per 100,000
    1998 --- 23.2 cases per 100,000   [182]

This decline of course has nothing to do with the vaccine. The vaccine came in 2002. But the figures still seem a little high, don't they? On closer inspection, reading the microprint footnote on that same page, we read:

 "Includes cases imported from outside the United States"

Huh? 'Cases imported from outside the United States'? We're not talking Beaujolais here. No one doubts that the vast majority of hepatitis A cases are foreign. A disease of poverty, filth, and malnutrition, the trick here is that global incidence of this disease was used to calculate the necessity for the vaccine in the US.

THE VACCINE ITSELF

Hepatitis A vaccine is made from **infected human connective tissue** cells. Not from just one guy, but rather each batch of vaccine is made from an infected mass of cells which had 1000 donors. (*Pediatrics*) [268] The cells are infected with hepatitis A virus, the agent presumed to be present in every case of hep A.

The agents are filtered, and attenuated with aluminum, formalin, and phenoxyethanol - a synonym for ethylene glycol – a component in antifreeze. (*PDR*, p1456) [244]

ALUMINUM AND FORMALDEHYDE

It is not just its connection with Alzheimer's that makes aluminum such a danger to human physiology. Aluminum can interfere with the formation and development of virtually any human nerve tissue, in a fully unpredictable fashion. [249, 216]

As for formaldehyde, exactly how much danger of cancer is an acceptable risk in the pure, perfect blood of a newborn? Cancer occurs first in just one cell. So where are the studies that prove that this "trace" of formaldehyde or antifreeze will not be sufficient to cause that first cell mutation that develops into cancer? **No vaccines are tested for carcinogenicity**. None of them. ([75] *PDR*)

THE DISEASE IS SAFER THAN THE VACCINE

Was it really necessary to introduce an infectious virus into the entire population of children in order to pretend to prevent a disease which is virtually nonexistent in the United States?

If the disease itself is mild and self limiting and confers true lasting immunity, wouldn't it be better for that very low number of people just to get the disease and forego the addition of carcinogens and neurotoxins into the common bloodstream?

More on Hepatitis A: see chapter at thedoctorwithin.com [181]

HEPATITIS B

Hepatitis B is an inflammatory liver disease, found most often among drug addicts. Most victims recover on their own within a few months, with no chronic liver disease. In 1991, however, the CDC and the AAP began including Hepatitis B vaccine for all infants. (p 172 [215])   Why?

Before 1991, hepatitis B vaccine was only given to high risk groups - health workers, drug users, those with multiple sex partners, and those with a history of the disease. The disease is transmissible from mother to infant, but if the mother tests negative, it is very unlikely that the infant will have multiple sex partners or be an IV drug abuser, know what I'm saying?

Especially within the first day of life. This is the type of common sense notion that gets overlooked when fortunes are to be made.

Efficacy? No long-term studies had been done before the vaccine was forced on the general population. (Neustaedter, p125) [215] The insert itself says that the vaccine was only monitored for **5 days** before it was released on the market! (Dunbar) [188]

Merck had been developing the Hep B vaccine since the early 1970s, and testing it on live populations of monkeys and humans. (p.244) [248] Formaldehyde, a carcinogenic 'inactivator' used in many vaccines, supposedly tones down the Hep B virus so that the vaccine hopefully doesn't give the person hepatitis.

But the real horror of Hepatitis B vaccine comes into focus when you find out that this mercury-laden vaccine is given on the first day of life. The EPA "safe" level of mercury is .1 micrograms per kilogram per day. For an adult, that is. As of 2004, one hepatitis B shot had 30 times that amount! - FDA *Hepatitis Control Report*, vol. 4, no. 21.   [274]

Side effects?   The CDC failed to mention any side effects in **8 million people** who received the vaccine before 1991. (p 175) [215] But a number of studies have documented the following adverse reactions to the Hepatitis B vaccine:

Guillain-Barre	**enlarged spleen**
demyelinating disease	**anaphylactic shock**
autoimmune reactions	**jaundice**

In a statement to Congress, Director of the Association of American Physicians and Surgeons Jane Orient, MD said that deaths and adverse reactions to hepatitis B vaccines are

"...vastly underreported, as formal long-term studies of vaccine safety have not been completed."   [190]

"...for most children the risk of a serious vaccine reaction may be 100 times greater than the risk of Hepatitis B."

As of 1999, the number of reported severe adverse reactions to the Hep B vaccine became higher than the actual number of cases of the disease itself! (*Townsend Letter*, Sep 2000, p 148) [183]

Hepatitis B vaccination was dropped from the mandatory school program in France in Oct. 1998 after 15,000 citizens filed a class action suit against the government. The reason: hundreds of neurological and auto-immune disorders. (Belkin) [260]

CHEERLEADING FOR HEPATITIS B VACCINE

There were at least 6 articles in the *New York Times* in 2008 in which the conclusion, always by some junior health writer, was that unvaccinated children pose a risk to the community at large, because they perpetuate disease.

On 1 Oct 08 the *NYT* ran a story titled "Study Links Hepatitis B And Cancer Of Pancreas." [68]

There was no actual study, nor did the article definitely link anything to anything. In a cursory review of data with cancer patients, they noticed a higher than normal history of hepatitis B among one group of cancer patients. The authors themselves claim no definite causality between the two conditions - it's just initially noteworthy. [69] This was an **epidemiological study**, which means it's not a study at all, just a first-draft data comparison. It's an idea for a study; that's all.

This confused essay of 1 Oct 08 made the unfounded statements:

"chronic hepatitis B ... Globally, is a major cause of liver cancer."

" ... A vaccine can prevent the infection and the cancer. But when an unvaccinated person develops a chronic infection, it cannot be cured, though antiviral drugs may help control it."

First of all hepatitis B may only become chronic 5% of the time. [266] *Merck* p 382]   It is chronic hepatitis that is associated with liver cancer, not the mild self-limiting variety, which is 90% of the cases with hep B. ([70] Jay Marks, MD)

Secondly, there is no proof of efficacy for a hepatitis B vaccine for any infection, as we have already seen above. **Nor can any vaccine prevent cancer. Or any infection!** Even the manufacturers of Hep B vaccine would never claim that it can prevent cancer - that is impossible. How then does a feature writer get away with making such a baroque claim in a national publication?

Third, when the unvaccinated contract any infection, they stand just as much chance of cure as anyone else. Being unvaccinated does not lower the immune system; in fact it's just the opposite.

The vaccinated, especially infants, have a much more difficult time fighting off infections, because of the immuno-suppressive nature of experimental attenuated agents and toxic adjuvants. Remember, **vaccines are not given for infections.** They never were, and no scientist ever made such an absurd claim.

Never a bastion of fourth estate ethics or responsible reporting, it has been apparent in recent years that the *NYT* has become a repository for sensationalistic copy, with a decreasing level of accountability, if not a mouthpiece for the drug industry. A quick look at the ads in any issue will illuminate their allegiance. In the business of casting aspersions and innuendo, things like reliability and fact checking go quietly by the wayside.

Assuming readers are getting dumber all the time, editors figure they don't really have to be accountable or verify what they say, since it's only about creating an impression, an instant impression as people speedscan the article on their way to wherever.

PARENTS RESPONSIBLE FOR HEP B REACTIONS

There's a related story every parent should read, especially those who think they're doing the right thing to vaccinate a newborn with the dangerous Hepatitis B shot. If the baby has a reaction, the parents are now the prime target for accusations of **Shaken Baby**! Not kidding - this happens all the time. Look at – ([6] Elber)

ROTAVIRUS

Rotavirus is a poorly understood illness of infants, usually involving a mild, self-limiting case of diarrhea. The biggest danger to the child is dehydration, but that occurs only in rare cases. The old name was **colic**, which for the majority of infants usually passes in a short time without complication. The few cases of death that result worldwide happen in the poorest locations on earth, where starvation and disease are common:

"90% of all deaths from the vaccine occur in Africa and Asia" [83] In the US there may be as few as 20 deaths per year, taking into account the most unhygienic environments, and including adults. [84]

Using global statistics to sell domestic vaccines is a common sales technique.   How the rotavirus vaccine became added to the schedule back in 1998 was more a matter of politics than of science. In the *Merck Manual* rotavirus infection is not described as a serious disease. Rotavirus is often found in asymptomatic infants. ([266], p 2173) It is so trivial a disease that the only recommended treatment before the vaccine came out was re-hydrating the infant. [266]

RotaShield was added to the mandated schedule in 1998. Then after so many complaints of a sometimes fatal disorder of the infant's bowel called **intussusception**, and other injuries following vaccination, the CDC quietly took RotaShield off the market in after only 11 months. (*Newsweek*, 13 Sep 99) [236]

Paul Offit, who was on the CDC Board of Advisors that approved rotavirus vaccine, admitted in Congressional hearing that he not only received benefits from the vaccine's manufacturer, Merck, but that he actually **owned the patent**! Asked if he thought that could be a conflict of interest, Offit made the condescending reply:

"I am a co-holder of a patent for a (rotavirus) vaccine. If this vaccine were to become a routinely recommended vaccine, I would make money off of that. ... am I biased? That answer is really easy: absolutely not."

"Is there an unholy alliance between the people who make recommendations about vaccines and the vaccine manufacturers? The answer is no." [317]

Offit has been receiving funding from Merck for the past 17 years for promoting rotavirus vaccines. He received one grant of **$350,000** from Merck to develop the rotavirus vaccine [89].

It's just business. Representative Dan Burton puts it like this:

"CDC routinely allows scientists with blatant conflicts of interest to serve on influential advisory committees that make recommendations on new vaccines," Burton told UPI. "... these same scientists have **financial ties**, academic affiliations, and vested interests in the products and companies for which they are supposed to be providing unbiased oversight."   [317]

ROTATEQ STEPS UP

After the 1999 RotaShield fiasco, it was almost inconceivable that they would try again. Yet in a fit of post 9/11 power politics, a new version of the vaccine was trotted back out in early 2007, with whirlwind approval by the FDA and introduction right back into the Mandated Schedule. Only it had a new name: **Rotateq**.

Rotateq's debut came with new reports of the same major side effect that occasioned the earlier vaccine being pulled 9 years before: - **intussusception**. This condition is sometimes fatal, and usually requires surgery. It was not even associated with the original disease, but only with the vaccines.

Other side effects of Rotateq: NVD, otitis media, pharyngitis, and bronchospasm.

The primary study of the clinical trials cited by Rotateq's manufacturer – Merck – was published in the *New England Journal of Medicine* in Jan 2006. [87] This study was funded by Merck, used Merck trial protocols, and was co-authored by the owner of the patent of both the original vaccine and the current version. The majority of the authors were listed at the bottom as being given financial perqs from Merck.

Rotateq wasn't much different from the old RotaShield, except for one additional viral strain and the fact that the testing was done on human infants, not monkeys. [244]

The vaccine made little difference:

   "Among the 9605 subjects in the detailed study (4806 in the vaccine group and 4799 in the placebo group), the rates of fever, vomiting, and diarrhea within 42 days after any dose were similar among vaccine recipients and placebo recipients.."

Serious adverse events were reported in 803 of 34,035 vaccine recipients (2.4 percent), with **24 deaths** in the vaccinated group.

The most common cause of death was **Sudden Infant Death** syndrome, which occurred in **seven** vaccine recipients.

Over and over the new sales pitch keeps talking about how the incidence of intussusception was nothing out of the ordinary, how the vaccine does not cause intussusception, etc. [87] With intussusception as the main reason the old vaccine was pulled 10 years ago, the authors thought they had to pacify and reassure the new market.

So it was astounding then that less than a month after being added to the Schedule, the FDA began warning the public of the exact same side effect from the new Rotateq, citing 28 new cases! [84]

   "The condition, called **intussusception**, is the same that led to the withdrawal of the first rotavirus vaccine eight years ago."

NEW PRODUCT, OLD MARKETING

RotaShield was probably the only vaccine in history that was not included in the *PDR*. Today it's virtually impossible to find any evidence that RotaShield ever existed.

RotaShield was slightly different from the new Rotateq. Rotashield was from human and monkey sources, whereas the newer Rotateq is from human and bovine sources. Outside of that, the song is pretty much the same with Rotateq – claims of 95% efficacy, completely safe, very necessary.

Infant colic is not something for which any vaccine is needed, let alone one as toxic and immunosuppressive as Rotateq.

AUTISM: A TRUE EPIDEMIC

The 1990s brought a new disease phenomenon – autism – which suddenly showed up in hundreds of thousands of normal 2 year olds. The child stopped developing, stopped responding, stopped learning and withdrew into this permanent condition of arrest. Most of them never speak and 75% of them are unable to ever live independently. The family is socially and financially devastated. The overall cost from the epidemic is measured in **trillions**.

Since the early 1990s autism has certainly met the definition of an epidemic, although both medical and popular literature can never use the words **epidemic and autism** in the same sentence.

In 1978, there were less than 1 in 10,000 autistics. Today the best estimate is **between 2 and 4 million**. There is no cure. Mainstream medicine refuses to acknowledge autism as an epidemic, and has steadfastly refused to look for a cause.

The CDC admitted to over half a million autistics by Apr 2006. [93] A better guess can be extrapolated from US Dept of Education statistics on child disability. [85] According to their charts, autism rose geometrically in all 50 states from 1993 - 2006. The chart shows average state increases of **1700%** looking at only 15% of total cases.

By 2009 HHS was estimating **1 in 91 children** with ASD. [324, journal *Pediatrics*]

In many areas of the US even higher incidence is reported: 1 in 67, and even 1 in 25!

Taking all reasonable sources into consideration, best total estimate for 2011 would be **2-4 million** autistics in the US. Yet the word epidemic is strictly forbidden in reference to autism.

The physical mechanism between vaccines and autism is clear:

   "Vaccines provoke an immune response to an antigen derived from a virus or bacteria. They can also contain adjuvants, which augment the antibody response and provoke inflammation throughout the body… as well as preservatives such as mercury.

 "Aluminum and mercury can enter the brain and remain for years, where they provoke **neuro-inflammation**. Inflammation during childhood can interfere with the normal mechanisms … leading to neurodevelopmental disorders such as autism."   [18, Deth]

With autism, the causative mechanism stems from **myelin defects**.

DANISH STUDY: MILLIONS FOR MISDIRECTION

A research project carried out in Denmark in 2003 and published in *Pediatrics* [321] – the ill-fated Madsen study – for years assured the world of the usual mantra with respect to thimerosal and vaccines: no possible connection. Since that time a thorough explosion of the fatally flawed study has been available on Scudamore's definitive site [323]. Nevertheless, up until recently the Danish study still served as a pivotal defense source for those clinging to the hope that the autism/mercury connection could be kept hidden.

No more. One of the principal co-authors of that study, Poul Thorsen, has now been indicted on a host of charges, including falsification of data, money laundering, etc. stemming from that original study. Not necessary to cite a particular reference here — just google the phrase 'Poul Thorsen indicted' and over 200,000 references will come up.

The study was funded by the CDC, and they want their money back. And they won't be citing the Danish study any longer in their defense of mercury. [323]

The unflinching refusal by FDA, CDC, US Dept of Health, NIH to fund legitimate clinical trials on a possible autism/vaccine connection has left it to independent researchers to try and find the true cause. What they have come up with, both in Congressional committees and independent research is overwhelming and incontrovertible evidence that the autism epidemic has

TWO PRIMARY VACCINE-RELATED CAUSES:

Mercury
MMR vaccine   [142, 110]

MMR vaccine does not contain mercury.

Mercury in vaccines is in the form of **thimerosal**.

Both causes have been widely explored. But never by mainstream science. The subject is verboten.

MEASLES - MUMPS - RUBELLA VACCINE

In the US, the MMR vaccine was added to the mandated schedule in 1978, approved after studies lasting only **28 days**. [147] We saw the sales pitch above. To this day, no medium or long-term safety studies of MMR have ever been done.

HERD IMMUNITY

As we were led down the path of MMR vaccination, 2000 centuries of herd immunity - natural immunity - were cavalierly tossed out the window. Before the vaccine, whoever got one of these mild diseases thereby got lifetime immunity. No longer. Instead, after a couple of decades of vaccination, we now see **atypical versions** of the original diseases: brand new adult disease forms. Manmade.

Herd immunity is far older than vaccines. Do not make the error of many pediatricians or 'journalists' who talk about herd immunity as though it refers to the immunity that proceeds from a large group of people being vaccinated. The calculated deception behind this common malapropism is that if you don't know what herd immunity is, you'll buy their illusion: that the unvaccinated child cannot take advantage of the herd who have been vaccinated. This is well thought-out propaganda. True herd immunity is a term which indicates that a disease has burned itself out within a population, as with plague, smallpox, typhus - every infectious disease in history. The herd has become immune. Natural selection. It has to do with nature, not with vaccines. Don't be fooled again.

Adults who get measles, mumps, or rubella for the first time have a much greater chance of death or serious complications. (Merck) [266] MMR vaccine may actually work to delay the onset past childhood; as a result, the adult versions are mutated forms of the original diseases. Which means that someone who got the disease as a child and who was thereby immune for life, **may not now be immune to the new atypical forms created by mass vaccines**.

MMR AND AUTISM

Forget everything you have heard about Andrew Wakefield.

About 1996, Wakefield a London surgeon / gastroenterologist noticed that autistic children had a severe bowel disorder. Wakefield began to do something that other doctors hadn't done - examine the children, starting with abdominal palpation, to feel for an obvious obstruction.

After a colonoscopy on each child, Wakefield noticed a pathology: large nodular bleeding masses within the child's colon.

The condition - **lymphoid nodular hyperplasia** – was unimaginably painful for the infant because these bleeding, swollen, infected nodules blocked the colon. The body would interpret the nodules as waste and attempt to pass them through. But since they were attached to the lining of the colon, a pathological folding up or telescoping of the colon would occur, which doctors call intussusception. Usually surgical, often fatal.

Wakefield began to call the new bowel disease **autistic enterocolitis**. This was quite a different thing from your average infant colic. The autistic colon had some unique features that appeared in virtually every case:

- inner lining of intestine blocked and inflamed
- lymphoid nodular hyperplasia
- specific viral infection
- autoimmune characteristics

What could make a two year old's colon attack itself?

VIRAL CONNECTION

Good question. A molecular biologist, John O'Leary PhD, was asking the same thing. O'Leary's contribution was a sophisticated sequencing technology (TAQMAN) that can distinguish one virus from another. In almost every autistic gut, they found measles virus - the virus from the measles vaccine component of the MMR shot. (Uhlmann) [155]

CAREER SUICIDE

At this point Wakefield made a career-defining statement. He merely suggested that perhaps a connection between autism and MMR vaccine deserved further study. [271] That was it. Suddenly he found himself the target for censure from the worldwide medical community. Too late he discovered his mortal sin: he had unintentionally maligned the Sacred Cow of medicine - vaccines. He then watched his brilliant career take that long slow swan dive, from which he has never recovered.

A lesser man would have apologized and backed off, like his co-authors did. Yet Wakefield, seeing a reasonable hypothesis that was being ignored by science, was undeterred. He saw the vital importance of such a discovery if it turned out he was correct.

PLAUSIBILITY: FIRST PIECE OF THE PUZZLE

Wakefield first asked: is it plausible for a viral agent like measles vaccine to be the cause of a neurological disorder like autism? Is there a recognized link between the gut and the brain? Nothing controversial here. Aspirin is absorbed into the bloodstream through the stomach, and cures headaches. Beer is absorbed through the bloodstream and alters mood. Prozac is taken into the digestive system and alters mood. Poisons we eat may damage parts of the brain which are necessary for survival.

Years ago, Chopra spoke of the brain chemicals that were found all through the digestive tract, sending constant information back and forth. (Chopra) [262] Psychoneuroimmunology, a huge field today, studies the sophisticated feedback mechanisms linking the immune system, the gut, and the brain.

ANOTHER PIECE OF THE PUZZLE

One of the world's leading autism research scientists Jeff Bradstreet, MD:

"... we propose a subset of genetically vulnerable children who **lack the ability to clear the vaccine strain of the virus** and that this is ... a direct cause of their symptoms." [114]

Why isn't NIH funding such an important hypothesis?

Wakefield shows graphs of the **US and UK 10 years apart** that were identical in tracing the skyrocketing incidence of autism just after the **MMR vaccine** was introduced:

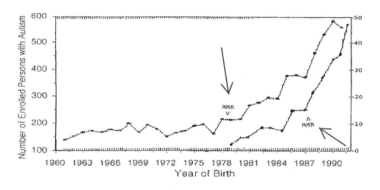

Left graph US 1978. Right graph UK 1988.   Fairly suspicious.

VIRAL INTERFERENCE

Doctors have a name for triple shot vaccines: **trivalents**. Wakefield wonders at the lack of science behind mixing 3 viral agents together in one triple shot vaccine cocktail like MMR without testing the mix. Viral agents have unpredictable effects upon each other. The random result of mixing together viral agents is called **viral interference**. It is discussed in more than 2000 journal articles. [147]   1+1+1 does not necessarily equal 3.

With measles/mumps/rubella vaccine - we have manmade strains of three infectious viruses thrown together. Not the naturally occurring disease strains, mind you, but manmade forms. Early researchers pointed out the necessity for further study. (Buynak,

1969 [265], Minayama - 1974) Later researchers reaffirmed that these viral interactions should be thoroughly studied with all triple shot vaccines. (Halsey)[198] To this day, that work has **never been done**. Looking at the current Schedule of vaccines we see no less than **seven triple shot** injections mandated for every American child. [26]

THE AUTOIMMUNE MEASLES VACCINE

V. Singh, PhD, a specialist who has studied hundreds of cases of autism, found that these children experienced an autoimmune episode, in which their own body began to attack the lining of the nervous system - **myelin** - analogous to the insulation of electronic wire in your computer. Singh: "hyper-immune response to the measles virus."   Such damage is a well-known effect of the mercury used in vaccines, as well as of the measles vaccine. No child is born with intact myelin.   Flawed architecture in the formative infant brain can result in virtually any childhood or adult neurologic disorder. [143]

Despite the massive denial and coverup from mainstream media and organized medicine in the past decade, thanks to Wakefield, Singh, Dan Burton, and a few others, here's what can be said of most autistics:

• normal early development
• regression to autism after vaccine
• a new GI pathology not found in normal children
• recurrent infections
• neurological symptoms characteristic of brain toxicity
• LN hyperplasia in the colon: as a response to virus
• immune deficiency/autoimmune characteristics

PROVE THEM WRONG

With all the billions available from the NIH for medical research, where are the parallel studies being done to disprove Wakefield? If his methods are wrong, duplicate them and discredit him once and for all. What if it turns out Wakefield is right? Isn't an epidemic that affects one infant in 67 worth studying?

Not one dime will ever be spent replicating Wakefield's experiments, but endless sums will be spent demonizing him. Why? Because every scientist knows what they will find: Wakefield would be found correct. There is an unarguable causal connection between MMR and autism. In fact, his findings have been corroborated 5 times by legitimate studies, which have been suppressed. [10] But the mid-1990s class action payouts by the tobacco industry – over $250 billion – would pale by comparison to settlements that would result from even a scintilla of admission about a link between autism and vaccines, especially from their two most toxic sources – thimerosal and MMR.

NEXT UP: MERCURY AND AUTISM

What is **mercury**? An elemental metal, liquid in its natural form, historically mercury was called quicksilver. Mercury is the **third most toxic substance known to man**. It is the most toxic nonradioactive metal. (Bernard) [180]

Scientists have known for decades that mercury is poison. But most study has been of mercury contamination of fish and from toxic spills. The mercury in vaccines, as we saw above, is in the form of **thimerosal** which is 49.5% mercury. This is **ethylmercury**, a manmade neurotoxin (nerve killer) that is far more toxic than inorganic mercury. (Koos) [283] Shot into a newborn's bloodstream on the very first day of life as part of the Hepatitis B vaccine, thimerosal is allowed to be in direct contact with brand new unformed tissues:

- intestine lining
- liver
- brain
- nervous system

Since 1997, the official mantra has been: there is no proof that thimerosal causes autism, or any other disease. But change just one word and it all shifts: there is abundant scientific proof that thimerosal can cause autism, and virtually any other neurological disorder as well.

WHAT DO THE MANUFACTURERS SAY?

Two manufacturers of thimerosal are **Eli Lilly** and **EMD Chemicals**. Here's what their own Safety Data Sheets state:

Eli Lilly: "Effects of Exposure: .. allergic dermatitis... mercury poisoning can occur.... Signs ... in adults are nervous system effects, including narrowing of the visual field and numbness in extremities. Exposure *in utero* and in children can cause **mild to severe mental retardation** and mild to severe motor coordination impairment. [132]

EMD Chemicals: "DANGER! POISON! MAY BE FATAL IF INHALED, ABSORBED THROUGH SKIN OR SWALLOWED. EYE AND SKIN IRRITATION. ... MAY CAUSE DAMAGE TO THE

FOLLOWING ORGANS: KIDNEYS, RESPIRATORY TRACT, SKIN, EYES, CENTRAL NERVOUS SYSTEM, EYE, LENS OR CORNEA. HARMFUL TO ENVIRONMENT IF RELEASED IN LARGE AMOUNTS. WARNING: This product contains a chemical known to the State of California to cause birth defects or other reproductive harm." [309]

So then, thimerosal clearly **can** cause autism. The carefully scripted "studies" and news releases always deftly sidestep this glaring admission by the manufacturers.

WHAT DOES MERCURY DO?

In her 2000 monograph - *Autism: A Unique Type of Mercury Poisoning* - Sally Bernard traces the history of mercury to its origins. Providing a shocking comparison of 2 conditions: mercury poisoning and autism, she notes that both diseases affect the same 6 systems:

gut	**muscle control**
brain	**immune system**
eyes	**speech**

Bernard shows a virtual one-to-one correspondence between the symptoms of autism and those of mercury poisoning. [180]

Since 1930 there have been 4 separate government agencies that have set toxicity levels for mercury. Amazingly, not one of them even considered the two greatest exposures that children have to mercury: thimerosal in vaccines and dental amalgams. [180]

CENTRAL NERVOUS SYSTEM

One of the most frequent complications of vaccinations "gone wrong" seems to be diseases of the central nervous system. It is easy to understand why in the case of children. No matter what presumptions we may employ, **children are not miniature adults**. Their nervous systems are not near complete. Nerve tissue is the most delicate and sensitive substance, arguably in the entire universe. The insulation around nerves - **myelin** - is not yet formed at birth. During its development, nerve tissue is exquisitely sensitive to minute changes in its biological environment. The presence of mercury in the blood can prevent normal nerve formation. (University of Calgary video [141])

Even minute traces. **There is no safe level**.

Inflammation and oxidative stress within the child's brain resulting from mercury can cause autism, or virtually any neurologic disease. [18, Deth] [334, Blaylock]

Theo Colborn clearly explains that a substance that may have been harmless to an infant at two years of age may effect a devastating, permanent glitch in the carefully orchestrated configuration of the central nervous system, if experienced at two months, or six months, or at one day. (p.113) [216]

ORGANIC VS INORGANIC MERCURY

Bernard shows that the reason thimerosal is a much more toxic form of mercury than one would get from eating open-sea fish has to do with the difficulty of clearing thimerosal from the blood. Thimerosal is **ethylmercury**, a manmade organic form which has a preference for nerve cells. Without a blood-brain barrier, an infant's brain and spinal cord are sitting ducks. Once in the nerve cells, mercury becomes tightly bound. It can accumulate there for years, like a time-release capsule, causing permanent degeneration of brain cells, in an unpredictable fashion. [180]

And this is how thimerosal can be the original and unidentifiable cause of virtually any neurological disease that mysteriously pops up later in life, with no way to prove it.

In living things, mercury is **bioaccumulative**. In man it is stored in fat cells, and persists year after year. [180]

SAFETY TESTS AND DOGS

Congressman Dan Burton got sort of miffed when he found out from government officials about their carelessness in monitoring mercury safety in vaccines for children during the past 8 decades:

> **"You mean to tell me since 1929 we've been using thimerosal and the only test that you know of is the one that was done in 1929, and every one of those people got meningitis and they all died?"** - Burton, 19 Jun 02 [154]

Eli Lilly, the inventor of thimerosal, did that test and hid the results, since they were getting the first thimerosal vaccines approved that year. [100]

Surrealistically, in 80 years there has never been another clinical test on thimerosal! - V. Williams [154]

Would anyone like to take a shot at explaining why in 1992 the

FDA found it necessary to take thimerosal out of dog vaccines but to leave it in children's? [154]

HOW MUCH MERCURY DO BABIES REALLY GET?

In an article in *Journal of the American Medical Association* in 1999, the EPA is quoted at setting .1mcg/kg/day as a maximum "safe" level of exposure to mercury. [198] (Halsey)   **For adults.** That's point-one micrograms per kilogram per day. Let's look at an FDA citation that interprets those safety levels in light of what an American child actually received by 2005:   [274]

   Day of birth: hepatitis B -   12 mcg mercury   30x EPA safe level

   At 4 months: DPT and HiB - 50 mcg   60x EPA safe level

   At 6 months: Hep B, Polio -   62.5 mcg   78x EPA safe level

Now EPA levels were talking about inorganic mercury, like from ocean fish, or broken thermometers, etc.   And they were also talking about safety levels for adults.

But thimerosal in vaccines is an **organic** form, logarithmically more bindable to human tissues. Especially brain cells.   [277]

And vaccines are given to infants.

Here's one reason why it's more toxic. From the *AAPS Journal*:

   "...mercury in vaccines is given by injection rather than by oral ingestion only makes the exposure levels worse because ...the distribution reached **several logs** higher concentration in organs following ...injections than via oral ingestion." [118]

Several logs? You mean exponentially by powers of 10?

DATA CORRELATING MERCURY WITH AUTISM

Authors who state there is no evidence of a connection between mercury and autism are talking nonsense. Here is a graph from the *Journal of American Physicians and Surgeons* which correlates mercury with autism: [118]

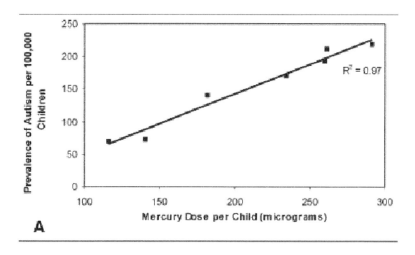

How much education do you need to read this chart? The more mercury, the more autism.

Research by Bradstreet et al. presented 9 Feb 2004 to the Institutes of Medicine hearings shows a

"direct association between increasing mercury from

thimerosal-containing   childhood   vaccines   and   neuro-development disorders in children." [113]

Because of overwhelming evidence, the study concluded that

   "mercury should be removed immediately from all biologic products."

That's exactly what the FDA said back in 1999 when it "asked" vaccine manufacturers to leave thimerosal out. Asked. CDC and APA joined the 'recommendation.' [127]

But thimerosal was never banned, nor can it ever be. As above, settlements. Class action. Banning it would be confirming its toxicity in vaccines. No hint of that must see the light of day.

BLOOD BRAIN BARRIER

The same blood that flows everywhere in the body also goes to the brain. Because of its unique requirements, however, brain tissue cannot be freely exposed to everything in the blood. So during adolescence we develop a mechanism for survival whereby only certain compounds are allowed to come into contact with the brain. This process of selective absorption is called the **blood-brain barrier.** (Guyton p 788) [200]

As for the harmful molecules kept out of the brain, doctors call such substances **neurotoxins**. That means they kill brain cells.

Here is a partial list:

- **aluminum**
- **mercury**
- **aspartame**
- **monosodium glutamate**
- **formaldehyde**   *- Excitotoxins, The Crazy Makers* [249]

The main reason that vaccines are so harmful for infants is the neurotoxicity of the additives on formative brain tissue. [334]

Unfortunately, babies are not born with a blood-brain barrier. (Blaylock, p.71) [249] It isn't complete until maturity. With direct access to the brain, such toxins have two effects:

- **kill existing brain cells**
- **prevent myelin and brain interconnections from forming**

Interconnections: now we're talking about the ability to learn. Association. Programming the new hard drive.

Certain areas of the brain, like the ones that allow a baby to walk, or to speak, or to learn – if these are damaged in the unprotected environment of the infant brain, the problem may go unnoticed for years. Later on when an impairment is noticed, doctors will be running around looking for some recent event. Too late. It's already over.

FOREIGN MERCURY

Other countries are not quite so blasé with their children's health: thimerosal was banned from vaccines 20 years ago in Russia, Denmark, Austria, Britain, Japan, and Scandinavia. [100]

CONGRESS LOOKS AT AUTISM

The House Committee on Government Reform looked at autism during 2000-2003. Under the leadership of Dan Burton, it wasn't the usual whitewash. Burton's grandson is autistic.

From Burton's opening statement in the hearings:

"Through a Congressional mandate to review thimerosal in medicines, the FDA learned that childhood vaccines, when given according to the CDC's recommendations exposed **over 8,000 children a day** in the United States to levels of mercury that exceeded Federal guidelines. Is there a connection between this toxic exposure to mercury and the autism epidemic?" [145]

THE SMOKESCREEN OF GENETICS

Watch how the word 'genetics' pops up when mainstream press or 'science' is talking about a disease for which no drug or procedure has yet been marketed. Since money can't be made by claiming to cure the disease, it is said to be 'genetic,' meaning that the disease comes from unpredictable, uncontrollable sources for which the patient is not responsible.

Autism is in this category. Since they don't have a drug cure yet, autism must be genetic.

V. Singh, PhD from the Utah State University explains why genetics is an impossible rationale for the autism epidemic: the kids are normal until two years old. Then they regress into the permanent brainfog of autism. That's simply not the way a genetic event manifests itself in a population. [143]

Secondly, noting the geometric rise between 1993 and 2007 - autism happened way too fast. [135] Mass genetic defects appear in a population over a much longer period of time than 9 years. **A fast genetic shift is a 1% increase over 100 years, not 1700% in 14 years**. [77]

Thirdly, there's **no such thing as a genetic epidemic**. (Yazbak [124])

Autism came out of nowhere in the last 20 years. If you think it can be explained away as a genetic condition, perhaps we could interest you in some prime real estate in south Florida. Or maybe a piece of the Boeing that hit the Pentagon.

Don't fall for this cheap trick of journalistic semantics.

PERMANENT DISABILITY

Even if the cause of autism were proven tomorrow and stopped dead in its tracks, autism would plague this country for decades to come. Like Burton says, these autistics aren't just going to die.

They are going to live on for years and years as a huge drain on parents and on our society – trillion$. And not just fiscally. As big money continues to do everything it can to prevent the cause of autism from being studied, thousands of new defectives are created year after year.

The government agencies responsible for monitoring and controlling diseases and medicine are the FDA, the NIH, and the CDC. Like most alphabet departments, in everyday operation, health often takes a back seat to politics and money concerns. All three agencies have shown a concerted effort in preventing the real cause of autism from being studied.

HHS is no better. Here's Dan Burton's opinion of them, from Congress 10 Dec 02:   [141]

"Officials at HHS have aggressively denied any possible connection between vaccines and autism. They have waged an information campaign endorsing one conclusion on an issue where the science is still out. This has significantly undermined public confidence in the career public service professionals who are charged with ... assuring the safety of vaccines and increasing immunization rates."

In HHS' own archives in their *Statement on Thimerosal* we read: "...among the symptoms of exposure include mental retardation in children, loss of coordination in speech, writing, gait, stupor, and irritability and bad temper progressing to mania." [171]

Sound anything like autism?

These agencies have consistently attacked the few researchers who are struggling unaided to uncover the etiology of this epidemic. Historically, organized medicine has rarely sought the true causes of disease. It focuses rather on marketing cures for disease, even if they don't work.

Just imagine - what if it's really true that the prime cause of autism turns out to be vaccines? Who would tell us? Vaccines are the Sacred Cow of medicine   As the introduction to a lifetime of dependence upon medicines, vaccines are above reproach, above criticism. How could vaccines - the crowning achievement of scientific medicine - be the cause of disease? This is the question that cannot be asked, the thought which cannot be entertained.

DR HALEY ON THIMEROSAL

One of the world's foremost experts on thimerosal toxicity is certainly **Boyd Haley, PhD**, chairman of UK's chemistry department. Here are just a few conclusions from this man who has spent years of study on the topic:

"the case against thimerosal is so dramatically overwhelming that only a very foolish or a very dishonest person with the credentials to understand their research would say that thimerosal wasn't the most likely cause of autism."

"You couldn't even construct a study that shows that thimerosal is safe. It's just too toxic... If you inject thimerosal into an animal its brain will sicken. If you apply it to living tissue, the cells die. If you put it in a Petri dish, the culture dies. ... it would be shocking if one could inject it into an infant without causing damage. " [133]

"A single vaccine given to a 6 pound newborn is the same as giving a 180-lb adult 30 vaccines on the same day."

WHY THIMEROSAL IS HERE TO STAY

On 2 Apr 04 a bill was introduced into Congress to ban all mercury from vaccines by 2006: HR 4169. [129]   Nice gesture, but only a footnote now.

Then in 2005, the manufacturers began voluntarily to remove thimerosal. There was getting to be too much criticism, too much attention, too much science that could no longer be ignored, even by the bovine mentality of the American public, that mercury is a poison and therefore cannot be a preservative. (Baskin [146])

After 80 years of overwhelming evidence proving its deadly effects and how it could cause autism, vaccine makers were now going to begin limiting or omitting thimerosal in vaccines. [244]   So they created a new illusion – don't worry, we're phasing thimerosal out.

Pediatricians, as well as the popular press, have been misleading parents for years, telling them that thimerosal was already gone from vaccines. And that's why most people think that thimerosal is no longer something they have to be concerned about.

HOW MUCH MERCURY IN VACCINES TODAY?

Despite the endless doubletalk we still read in everyday media and in various government papers about the decreases in vaccine thimerosal, here are the actual current figures of allowable mercury in today's vaccines, hidden in a chart at the very bottom of the FDA's own webpage on thimerosal, as of 14 Mar 2008:

DTaP	.3 mcg	
DT	25 mcg	
Td	8.3 mcg	
TT	25 mcg	
Hep B	1 mcg	
Hep A	1 mcg	
Influenza	25 mcg	[71]

A 2008 report to the state of California admitted that **trace levels of mercury were expected in all vaccines**:   [325, Schechter]

"After analyzing autism client data from the California Department of Developmental Services, researchers concluded that the data "do not show any recent decrease in autism in California despite the exclusion of more than trace levels of **thimerosal** from **nearly all childhood vaccines**."

Why on earth would they phase it out? Thimerosal has never been made illegal, nor will it ever be. That would be like the American Dental Association outlawing amalgam fillings. These poisons betoken the very essence of the respective professions. The FDA never forced the issue, never banned mercury. Since 1930, the FDA has never done its job, has never protected people from this neurotoxin. Infested as it is with top lawyers and execs from the industry it pretends to regulate, the FDA cannot end thimerosal.

In addition, old vaccines can always be shipped to poor nations as emblems of American good will. [100]

THE KENNEDY REPORT

So in 80 years the FDA never protected the public from thimerosal. Since the early 90s the FDA has known that over 8000 children every day were being exposed to levels of mercury that far exceeded Federal guidelines. [145] But thimerosal is still legal.

Many became nervous with the June 2005 report on mercury by **Robert F. Kennedy Jr**: *Deadly Immunity*. [100]   The reader is directed to the entire report, accessible online. Kennedy reveals a few of the more egregious industry misdeeds of the past 15 years:

 - the secret 2000 meeting of scientists, regulators and vaccine reps in **Simpsonwood, Georgia** to discuss overwhelming new research proving a link between mercury and autism

- the bad judgment in suddenly adding 3 mercury vaccines for infants in 1991:   hepatitis B, hemophilus B, and DPT.

- the 15-fold increase in autism which directly followed

- the incontrovertible evidence from the world's leading toxicologists that thimerosal in the mid 90s created the epidemic of autism

- after the research was presented, instead of discussing the best ways to alert the public to the new dangers, the group spent the remaining time figuring out ways to **cover it up**

One concrete result of the meeting: the CDC commissioned a cover study from the IOM, which was completed in 2004. That study deliberately withheld all the shocking new research they had just uncovered, and actually turned it over to a private company, AHIP, in order to sidestep Freedom of Information accessibility. [100]

INSTITUTES OF MEDICINE LOOKS AT THIMEROSAL

On 9 Feb 04, the IOM, a branch of the National Academy of Sciences, at the behest of CDC, convened in order to lay to rest once and for all the thimerosal controversy. They invited 13 of the world's leading scientists on neurotoxicology to come to Washington and present data about an association between autism and thimerosal.

Reviewing the audio files of that meeting, available on the IOM's website [110] the listener gets a first-hand view of government. As one scientist after another brilliantly summarized years of research in his allotted 20 minutes, leaving little doubt of the causal association between mercury in vaccines and brain injury, the contradiction could not be ignored: with all this scientific evidence, how can the mantra that we kept reading about no proof, no proof, continue to be evoked? Here is a preponderance of evidence linking thimerosal not only with autism, but with virtually any neurological disorder.

OVER THE TOP

Even with the outcome pre-ordained by CDC, [100] it was a shocking surprise that in defiance of the deluge of evidence presented that day proving the contrary, IOM's formal conclusion was that there was still "no proven link" between autism and thimerosal.   [70]

Where they really went over the top, however, was when "IOM declared the case closed and – in a startling position for a scientific body – recommended that **no further research be conducted** [!]"

Summarizing the day's testimony, perhaps the most cogent statement came from Mark Geier, MD PhD, a leading authority on genetics:

  "This is about as proven an issue as you're going to see.. what is occurring here is a cover-up under the guise of protecting the vaccine program. If we're not convinced thimerosal isn't causing autism, I recommend that we spend $10 or $20 billion to find out what is causing it. Nobody's doing that." [105]

MAKING AUTISM AN INDUSTRY

The race to market autism as a cottage industry has attracted every MLM, health supplement, magic bullet, and fringe modality known to man, each one claiming to "cure" autism. Most of the seminal autism awareness groups metamorphosed into MLMs marketing cures. Since the money's in the cure, they've stopped asking where the epidemic came from. Don't worry - our doctor's protocols work, they hawk. Some of the contenders include

DMSA	**EDTA**
taurine	**carnosine**
herbal chelation	**alpha lipoic acid**
hyperbaric therapy	**transfer factor**

Some of these remedies have actually shown improved behavior on some scale or other. Some, like oral chelation, part of the 60 Day Program, actually do remove mercury from an infant's delicate physiology. [31] But isn't that the wrong question? Shouldn't we be asking how to prevent infants from exposure to these neurotoxins? Autism will never be acknowledged as an epidemic until a pharmaceutical drug or procedure is claimed as a cure.

A creditable summary of autism research today can be found on the website ageofautism.com [120] For autism detox protocol: [56].

GOING DOWN

No amount of creative writing can make the prospects for the future of autism in America look bright. Autism is usually permanent, no matter what the MLMers say. Although there are some effective programs [56] rarely will a vaccine damaged child recover and be 100% normal again.

Risk / benefit studies have never been done for any vaccines. Realizing this one simple fact, blindly accepting the dictates of the Mandated Schedule of vaccines puts the child in harm's way. Until parents start doing their homework on vaccines, it's inevitable we'll continue to mass produce thousands of permanently defective citizens year after year, for decades to come. [M. Lahey MD]

THE DEATH OF A CHILD

Before we overintellectualize the minutiae of the autism phenomenon here, let's step back a minute and consider what these parents actually experience.

At some point, most of us have watched an infant develop into a toddler and become a little human being. One of our highest joys is to see the various stages and milestones the child reaches, about the details of which we have probably bored our friends senseless. To play with a little one every day and watch the miracle of their discovery as their light grows daily brighter is not just one of our greatest joys, but is it not one of the main purposes of human life?

Got the set-up here? OK, so now imagine that after 2 years of carefully nurturing a child all day every day, with all the rewards and sacrifices that entails, suddenly all at once - click – the light goes out, the child stops responding, stops smiling, stops learning, and soon doesn't even recognize you. And he's not just sick – it's permanent. Forever. Can't unboil a hardboiled egg, and all that. Another liability.

Now the whole contract changes – now it's a one-way street. You still have to care for the child, but now there's nothing coming back your way – no response, no interaction, no love, no promise for the future. And after a long time you have to try your best to keep telling yourself it's not just some lab experiment. This is your child.

Take a second and imagine your child like that.

The most common lament of the parents, when they finally learn about the vaccine/autism connection, is "I wish I'd known." They all say the same thing: "I wish I'd known."

So that's what this book is then – a chance to know. Beforehand. But why would anyone study something until they need to? And there we have the worst tragedy of all – they need to know before they vaccinate.

PREVNAR

Since its addition to the Schedule in 2002, the Prevnar (PCV) vaccine has been surrounded by controversy. Prevnar contains elements of Strep pneumoniae and diphtheria bacteria, and is marketed as protection for otitis media and bacterial meningitis.

The first and most striking problem with Prevnar is the claim that it protects against **otitis media**, which is usually a simple earache. Practically all babies get temporary earaches, which are mild and self-limiting and resolve in a day or two. Even the 2007 *PDR* cites 90% as the figure for infant earaches. [244]

It may be surprising to review the definition of otitis media: "a visually abnormal tympanic membrane suggesting effusion" [244] (2007, p 3468) That means looking in the baby's ear, the ear drum appears red. This can happen after crying. There's no culture, no blood test, nothing besides looking in the ear necessary to diagnose the commonplace "otitis." Inflammation, not infection.

So why would violating a child's bloodstream with a vaccine be necessary to prevent such a mild condition?

Are there any side effects from such a marginally important vaccine? Here's a partial list, according to the manufacturer:

fever	**anaphylactic shock**
seizure	**hives**
heart failure	**gastroenteritis**
rash	**thrush**
asthma	**choking**
pneumonia	**conjunctivitis**
otitis media	- 2007 *PDR* p 3468 [244]

Wait a minute. Otitis media as a side effect of the vaccine? Wasn't that what the vaccine was for? And pneumonia? Is it a surprise that injecting healthy kids with *Strep pneumoniae* might cause pneumonia? And look at all the other serious side effects.

As we read through the manufacturer's description of the original clinical trials, he states that the subjects were receiving all other standard vaccines at the same time. So how many of these other vaccines list *otitis media* as a side effect? Answer: **5**.

Does that mean we needed this new vaccine to take care of a side effect from other vaccines? Looks like it. The only way this study would have been legitimate would have been if the control group were unvaccinated.

By the way, there were **12 deaths** among the original subjects. [244]

The next amazing part of the sales job for Prevnar is the claim of protection against **bacterial meningitis** – an extremely rare disease in the US. The 2007 *PDR* claims that the incidence is "7 per 100,000" ([244] p 3463) and cites a source from a study written up in the 2 Oct 1997 *New England Journal of Medicine* [169]. But looking at the actual figures cited in the *NEJM* study itself, one finds they are claiming less than **1 case per 100,000** of bacterial meningitis. ([169], page 970) Guess the *PDR* sales force figure no one would actually look up the sources they cite, which generally is true. We can learn two things here:

1. *PDR*'s sources can't necessarily be trusted, and
2. the incidence of bacterial meningitis is **7x rarer** than they claim.

PROVEN EFFICACY

Does the Prevnar vaccine work? This subject is addressed head-on by a very thoroughly researched article entitled ***Prevnar : a critical review of a new childhood vaccine***, by British educator Michael Horwin. [170] The original clinical trials on Prevnar resulted in only a **7% reduction in earaches** from the vaccine. That's the highest benefit they're can claim for Prevnar – a vaccine for simple childhood earache, with all the above dangerous side effects, that may only work 7% of the time.

QUID PRO QUO

Horwin also goes into a detailed analysis of the financial entanglements between FDA advisory committees who approved Prevnar and WyethAyerst, the manufacturer. He shows how the most visible proponents of Prevnar, the doctors who do the world lecture tours and have huge research funding and get coverage in medical publications - the specifics of the financial incentives they reap.   After a few minutes reading those sweetheart deals, the overall picture comes into focus quite nicely. [170]

CANCER AND INFERTILITY

The standard cancer disclaimer sentence appears in the manufacturer's 2007 documentation for Prevnar: "**has not been evaluated for carcinogenic potential or impairment of fertility**" ([244] p 3467). Meaning that they don't even know whether or not this unnecessary vaccine causes cancer or may render the child sterile or infertile in adulthood.

The final shocker is that the clinical trials done for Prevnar were for otitis media, not for meningitis. As far as meningitis is concerned, the *PDR* doesn't even claim efficacy; and yet all the CDC's promo literature recommends the vaccine for meningitis, in the absence of supporting science.   All that misrepresenting of meningitis statistics cited above is smoke and mirrors. So even though Prevnar is marketed by the pediatric sales force across the US as protection against otitis media and meningitis, the manufacturer never cites any studies actually performed for meningitis. It's an unfounded claim, a marketing technique.

It is astounding that when Prevnar was first introduced into the

Mandated Schedule, they started with 4 doses: at 2, 4, 6 and 12 months. And the two month dose is given on the same day along with 5 other vaccines! That remains the current Mandated Schedule dose.

Japanese are apparently a little less blasé about Prevnar than we are. In Mar 2011, both Prevnar and *H. influenzae* vaccines were banned in the entire country after **6 children died**. [1] That story was barred from American media and only carried in Europe, Asia and Canada.

Try asking any American parent what either of those vaccines is for. Go ahead. Both are still on our Schedule: 7 shots.

THE BIRTH OF THEORETICAL DISEASES

The Prevnar vaccine marked a departure in the philosophy of vaccine mandating: vaccines for theoretical diseases. In the past, vaccines were claimed to be necessary to prevent standard infectious diseases which were supposedly caused by known pathogens: MMR, DPT, hepatitis, smallpox. But in the post 9/11 world, it seems that diseases no longer have to be real to require a vaccine. All that is necessary now is to label and then market a threat. Any threat.

Like temporary redness of the eardrum.

H P V: THE FIRST CANCER VACCINE

It was inevitable. In the post 9/11 marketing frenzy questing for more and more bugs and diseases to make vaccines against, what could be a more promising candidate than the second highest cause of death in the US?

Cancer of the cervix has been on a gradual upswing during the past 3 decades, now affecting some 12,000 American women, 4,000 of whom die each year. (CDC, [250])

In the 1970s, herpes simplex virus was proposed as a possible cause, but that hypothesis was soon abandoned after epidemiological studies proved inconclusive. In the 1980s the next candidate suggested as the missing link was **human papilloma virus**. [319]

Before we continue, a word here about epidemiological studies.

EPIDEMIOLOGICAL STUDIES

also called **population studies**, are the poor cousin of true clinical trials. They are not controlled studies done under set scientific conditions, but rather attempts at verifying a hypothesis by counting the incidence of a certain disease within a certain population. The problem is that results from epidemiological studies are subject to widespread interpretation, depending on who's doing the counting, who decides the criteria for what gets counted, who publishes the results, etc. For this reason, epidemiological studies can be used to "prove" two opposite hypotheses. Simply put,

Epidemiological studies are intrinsically unable to uncover causal mechanisms [18, Deth]

In the exploding vaccine industry today, epidemiological studies are quickly becoming the standard to validate our need for more vaccines, because they're faster, cheaper, and capable of supporting practically any required outcome.

So, once herpes was ruled out, the new population studies then proposed human papilloma virus as a cause of cervical cancer, since that vaccine was in development.

The first problem is that there are over 100 strains of HPV, only a few of which are even theoretically linked with cervical cancer. [318] In addition, HPV is present in at least half the normal population, [318] almost never causing any disease or problems whatsoever. Indeed, HPV has never been conclusively proven as a the sole pathogen for any disease.

HPV AND CANCER

Now in any cancer, we're talking about a normal cell that mutated and then began to make copies of itself, unchecked.

The creators of the HVP/cancer mythology are pretending that the HPV came along, attacked some normal cells and mutated those cells and caused them to begin replicating themselves out of control. And that this is happening on a mass scale even though we just discovered it. And worse, that a vaccine can neutralize that type of attack on normal cervix cells.

Scientifically, what they're proposing is ludicrous.

Few scientists have a better grasp of the proposed virus/cancer model than Berkeley's Peter Duesberg PhD. In tracing the history of the HPV/ cervical cancer story, Duesberg explains why HPV is such an unlikely cause of any cancer:

"no set of viral genes is consistently present or expressed in human cervical cancers. [319]   ... **HPV does not replicate in the cancer cells**."

So if the mutated cervical cancer cells are not mutating because of abnormal viral genes being spliced into a normal cell, how could HPV be causing this cancer? Duesberg again:

"the **"hit-and-run" mechanism** of viral carcinogenesis was proposed. It holds that neither the complete [virus], nor even a part of it, needs to be present in the tumor. Obviously, this is an unfalsifiable, but also an unprovable, hypothesis." [319]

All that has ever been shown is that HPV is sometimes present in cervical cancer tissue, but it's also present in half the normal population. The causality has never been demonstrated.

There is a total lack of evidence that cervical cancer appears in women with HPV more often than in women without it. [319] And yet this will be the focus of the vaccine: to pretend to eliminate this ubiquitous virus from the body.

THE NEW HPV VACCINE

The original phrase used by Merck to link HPV with cervical cancer was "there is a strong connection." ([266] p 1964)

How that phrase got transformed to 'is the cause of' in two years time is more a matter of marketing than of science.

The HPV vaccine had been in the Merck pipeline for years, finally getting FDA approval in 2006. [80]   Merck's HPV vaccine is called

Gardasil.

What's in it? According to Merck's own data, the vaccine is made from "virus-like particles" from four strains of HPV. ([244] p 1984.) With no clinical studies proving it, HPV is cited by Merck in the *Physicians Desk Reference* as the cause of "over 70%" of cervical cancer cases.

The theory is that these virus-like particles will trigger the body to make antibodies that will be able to prevent the full-on natural strains of HPV from getting a foothold. For a year, anyway.

The Merck insert for Gardasil makes this unequivocal statement:

> "HPV causes squamous cell cervical cancer."

We've already learned above that such is not the case.

The market that Merck decided on was **12 year old girls**, with the unfounded pretext that HPV is sexually transmissible. We might as well get it at the start, went the ruse. The vaccine may be given now to 9 year olds. [318]

EXTRAVAGANT DEMANDS ON CREDIBILITY

With other vaccines for viral diseases, such as MMR, hepatitis B, and polio, what has never made sense scientifically is that the vaccines do not contain the original wild virus that occurs in nature and supposedly causes the disease. Instead the vaccine contains a **manmade mutation** of the natural virus that is claimed to be able to confer immunity by triggering the body to produce antibodies to the original disease. Now that was bad enough, since the vaccines are lab versions of the original microbes. But what they're asking us to believe about HPV is simply a flight of fancy. [88]

All physiology and immunology textbooks describe the triggering of immunoglobulin production as an extremely specific sequence, resulting in specific antibodies. [200, 320] They don't talk about cousins of viruses or particles from viruses being able to trigger the precise antibodies to the virus itself. Such a claim is brand new. How could any real immunity come from vaccines like these, even if the viruses were the causative agents of disease?

The second monster impediment to credibility is that the average age for cervical cancer is **50 years**. (*Merck Manual* p 1964 [266]) But the schedule mandates Gardasil to 12 year olds. And the manufacturer is only claiming efficacy for a year. So using their own statistics, this makes the vaccine worthless in the long run, because by the time most females need immunity, it will have worn off long ago.

A risk factor in cervical cancer that has been clearly established is the lifetime number of sexual partners: the more partners, the more likely the disease. ([266] p 1964) So who has more, 12 year olds or 50 year olds? Even if the vaccine worked, statistically it should be given to women in their late 40s. Why don't they do that? Here's the reason:

The vaccine's "safety and efficacy not been evaluated over 26" years of age. (2007 *PDR* [244] p 1987)

Oh, OK. Well, guess we better give it to the young girls then, even though they don't get the disease...

Anybody want to take a shot at why the vaccine is routinely given also to boys? For the first five years the FDA didn't recommend the vaccine for boys, despite the millions in research Merck had spent:

"The ACIP stopped short of recommending HPV vaccination of adolescent boys" (Kim [12])

But most clinics never caught the distinction and vaccinated both boys and girls. Finally in Feb 2011 they came up with a rationale, out of thin air: the HPV vaccine should be given to boys in order to prevent genital warts.

HPV VACCINE FOR BOYS

Approved in 2006 supposedly to prevent cancer of the cervix, HPV vaccine has been given indiscriminately to boys as well for the past 5 years. Nobody ever asked why. People finally began to notice it in 2010, and an unproven, untested rationale began to appear in pop media – that the HPV vaccine also prevented genital warts in boys. What a serendipitous coincidence – this vaccine that we have been claiming all this time will prevent cancer of the cervix in 12 year old girls, suddenly now this vaccine has the added value of preventing genital warts in 12 year old boys. And we just found out. How convenient then that they can both get the same vaccine on shot day!

This is the level of logic that the undiscerning public accepts as sensible – nothing coincidental about it. Even though there had been no studies of the vaccine and genital warts in boys, suddenly they're claiming its efficacy. So *NEJM* took up the bit in Feb 2011 with 2 new articles to prove the connection. The tone for the study is set in the second paragraph: [13, Giuliano] on p 401:

"The primary objective was to show that the HPV vaccine reduced the incidence of external genital lesions related to HPV"

Excuse us, but isn't the objective of any new clinical study to test a hypothesis? At least pretend like you're not merely providing the required evidence for your employers. Of course studies are done by the manufacturers who are attempting to prove a vaccine's effectiveness, but most have the good sense to at least simulate to be finding out whether it works or not.

Not surprising is the conflict of interest disclosure section at [13] in which almost all of the authors admit that they are either employees of Merck or have received financial rewards for doing the study.

The two 'new' studies are actually not new at all but just re-writes of data from 2004-2008. The old studies had no value until they were found to provide data for the new assignment: prove that the HPV vaccine prevents genital warts in boys. Which conclusion Merck's employees deliver, just as they were paid to do.

SIDE EFFECTS OF HPV VACCINE

Let's start with the ones cited by Merck:

fever	nausea	pharyngitis
dizziness	NVD	bronchospasm
Gastroenteritis	appendicitis	PID
upper respiratory infection		

- 2007 *Physicians Desk Reference* [244] p 1987

Additional side effects discovered later include **loss of**

consciousness, loss of vision and seizures. (Lopes, [79]) And oh yes, **paralysis**.

The British media began to report still other effects of Gardasil, like the **30 deaths**, which American media never mentioned. [86]

An additional symptom from the HPV shot is **Guillain Barre** syndrome, an autoimmune condition resulting in paralysis. There have been several such cases both in the UK and the US, including a high profile case in Oct 2008 of a 12 year old British girl who collapsed 2 days after the HPV shot and was subsequently paralyzed from the waist down. [86] Her first symptoms came on within 30 minutes. Again, no US media.

CARCINOGENICITY

Can the vaccine itself cause cancer? That's a fair question – we're talking about a vaccine that they're claiming prevents cancer by imitating a pathogen that itself causes cancer, right? So wouldn't we want to be fairly secure that this vaccine wouldn't cause cancer? Here's what the manufacturer states:

Gardasil "... **not been evaluated for carcinogenicity or impairment of fertility.** (2007 [244] p1986)

Wonderful. They want to vaccinate all American 12 year olds with a new vaccine for cancer and they don't even know for sure whether or not it causes cancer, or makes the recipients infertile.

Yeah, sign my kids up for that one, both boys and girls.

HPV VACCINE PROJECTED PROFITS

Gardasil is a 3 shot series at $360. [78]

   "The vaccine is expected to reach **$1 billion** in sales next year, ... could make Gardasil ...within five years, sales of more than **$4 billion**, according to Wall Street analysts." [80]

THE REAL QUESTION

Again, the whole story of HPV vaccine is much more twisted than we're representing here. The reader is invited to follow up the above cited sources. [41,11,79] Rarely has such a calculated, systematic misrepresentation of fact been attempted in which data is so obviously manipulated, issues so deliberately obscured, and financial interests so obsequiously served.

With the uncertainty about the safety and efficacy of the HPV vaccine, the certainty of the side effects, the prodigious economic upside to global dissemination irrespective of its scientific merits, the absence of long-term studies, and the ludicrous "religious /ethical/equality" media controversy smokescreen designed to distract us from the underlying scientific issues, is this really a vaccine you want to try out on your innocent little 9 yr old?

FDA ACCOUNTABILITY: MAKE MINE AN 'INCOMPLETE'

The members of the FDA who decide which vaccines get approved make up the Advisory Board (ACIP). In the Congressional investigation on vaccines, Rep. Dan Burton found out that financial statements of Advisory Board members were "incomplete." [141]

Noting that this is the only branch of government that allows incomplete financials, Burton called the Advisory Board's sweetheart arrangements with the vaccine manufacturers a "violation of the public trust." This includes **70%** of Advisory Board members who **admit to** owning stock in vaccines, owning patents on vaccines, and accepting salaries and benefits as employees of the drug companies both before and after their tenure on the Committee. [190, 317]

FOX GUARDING THE CHICKEN COOP

With a staff of 8000, the FDA exerts control over anything that is sold as a food or a drug in this country. This covers **one out of every four dollars** spent in the US. (Kessler [174]) Are we talking power and influence here? Or the potential for gifts and favors?

The words of ex-FDA Commissioner Dr. Herbert Ley echo today:

   "People think the FDA is protecting them. It isn't. What the FDA is doing and what the people think it's doing are as ... night and day. [299]

   "First, it is providing a means whereby key individuals on its payroll are able to obtain both power and wealth through granting special favors to certain groups that are subject to its regulation...For a price one can induce FDA administrators to provide protection from the FDA itself.

   "Secondly, ...cartel-oriented companies in the food and drug industry are able to use the **police powers of government to harass or destroy their free-market competitors**."

Any doubts about the FDA's true agenda, locate the one hour video [292] where Dr Stan Burzynski tells the story of how the FDA persecuted him for years about his life's work – the discovery of **antineoplastins**. This cancer injection resolves a high percentage of many incurable cancers, and has no side effects.   After continually suing Burzynski in court for imaginary transgressions, the FDA took the proprietary information Burzynski had provided for his defense and then literally **stole his patents**! Even though radiation and chemo have practically a zero % chance of success, antineoplastin therapy can only be used after these ineffective, potentially fatal remedies have been tried first. FDA doesn't want to cut into the chemo/radiation mega-industry. This isn't even the tip of the iceberg—before consenting to any cancer therapy, you have to find this DVD. [329]

Back in 2000, *USA Today* ran a series that took a hard look at the FDA. A few of their findings: [330]

- there are over 300 expert advisors on 18 advisory committees,
- making decisions on the approval of drugs and vaccines
- at least **54%** of them are being paid by the drug manufacturers
- since 1998, more than **800 conflict of interest** waivers have been issued to the various experts
- examples of conflicts: **stock ownership, consulting fees, research grants, spouses' employment and payments for speeches and travel**

POP QUIZ

How many drugs does the FDA test per year? Go ahead, guess. 10,000? 500? Give it your best shot. Ready for the answer? None. The FDA tests no drugs and no vaccines. They're a regulating agency, not a testing agency.

So just where do they get all their information about the testing that has been done on a new drug or vaccine? From the drug manufacturer! It's true. The FDA relies on the research data provided to it by the entities in line to make the most profit from the approval of the drug.

REVOLVING DOOR: FDA, CDC AND VACCINE INDUSTRY

Is CDC any more trustworthy? On 21 Dec 09 Julie Geberding, former CDC Director was named president of Merck, one of the world's largest vaccine manufacturers. [23] Throughout the 2009 swine flu game, did the CDC ever take any action on vaccines that did anything except promote their sale?   [32]

Or Klaus Stohr, head of WHO epidemiological all through Avian flu days, now a top exec with flu vax maker Novartis... On and on.

DOCTORS WHO DON'T VACCINATE

Because they know the information in this book, many MDs do not vaccinate their kids, but cannot say anything in public without threatening their licenses. [303]

Jane Orient MD is the Director of the American Association of Physicians and Surgeons. This group has gone on record that:

"vaccines... use school children as research subjects... without informed consent, in violation of the Nuremberg Codes.

"We suspect financial ties between vaccine manufacturers and medical groups such as the AMA and the American Academy of Pediatrics, which endorse the vaccine..." [190]

INCENTIVE GRANTS

Why would the school nurse care whether or not your kids are vaccinated? Why would she lie about exemptions? Ever wonder that? It's only money. The more kids get vaccinated, the more money that state gets from the fed:

"In an effort to improve state performance in reaching national immunization goals, the Senate Appropriations Committee ... in 1993 ... set aside... **$32 million** annually from the state infrastructure awards for incentive grants.

"These funds are distributed to the grantees [states] **according to their levels of immunization** coverage." [308]

Incentive grants comprise at least **24 percent** of the total grant awards to the states from the fed. [308]

"The federal government pays the state a bonus of **$100 for every fully vaccinated child.**." - *U.S. Newswire* [307, 308]

In the 2011 House bill in California to enforce vaccines among 7th graders, the author of the bill came right out and stated the reason for enforcing the shots:

"... bill author Sen. Christine Kehoe, D-San Diego, said the loss in attendance-based funding could amount to **$100,000 for some schools**." [333]

Attendance based funding – that's the phrase. Parents, you got that? Schools get federal money based on the percent of vaccinated children they can prove. That's why all the laws and monitoring.

MORE DOCTORS WHO DON'T VACCINATE

Mendelsohn, Phillips, Scheibner, Hay, Null, Blaylock, and others like them conclude that vaccinations generally should be avoided:

"The greatest threat of childhood diseases lies in the dangerous and ineffectual efforts made to prevent them through mass immunization. Much of what you have been led to believe about immunization simply isn't true. If I were to follow my deeper convictions, I would urge you to reject all inoculations for your child.

"There is no convincing scientific evidence that mass inoculations can be credited with eliminating any childhood disease. If immunizations were responsible for the disappearance of these diseases in the U.S., one must ask why they disappeared simultaneously in Europe, where mass immunizations did not take place."   [241] Robert Mendelsohn, MD

Australian researcher Viera Scheibner, PhD, after researching more than 60,000 pages of medical literature on vaccination:

"Immunizations, including those practiced on babies, not only did not prevent any infectious diseases; they caused more suffering and more deaths than has any other human activity in the entire history of medical intervention. It will be decades before the mopping-up after the disasters caused by childhood vaccination will be completed. All vaccinations should cease forthwith and all victims of their side effects should be appropriately compensated." [239]

Françoise Berthoud, MD from Switzerland:

"As a concerned pediatrician, I can arrive at only one conclusion. Unvaccinated children have by far the best chance of enjoying marvelous health. Any vaccination at all works to cripple the chances of this end."

From 100 years ago, Dr Raspail:

"Are we not poisoning humanity in small doses? It is diabolical that we are inflicting all these infections that have assaulted human beings at one time or another. It is stupefying, this arrogant introduction into the blood of a cocktail of germs when for the slightest surgical operation we wage unremitting war against them." [302]

From 150 years ago, pre-eminent French scientist **Dr Antoine Bechamp**:

"Bacteria and viruses do not cause disease and therefore serums and vaccines can neither prevent nor cure disease." [157]

There are dozens of other doctors who don't believe in any vaccines for their own children or their patients. An extensive list is located at whale.to – a comprehensive vaccine website from the UK [292]. There are tens of thousands of US parents today who don't vaccinate their children.

EXEMPTIONS: MANDATED VS. MANDATORY

An imposing system of disinformation is in place with regard to what parents are systematically told regarding school vaccinations. All they hear is that unless their child gets his shots, he will not be allowed to go to school. This is simply not true.

Mandated means that there are laws about something. **Mandatory** means you have to do something or other. Two entirely different concepts. Vaccines are mandated, but they are not mandatory, as school officials like to pretend.

No matter what you may read in newspapers and magazines, or what the school nurse may say, in most states your child can get into school without being vaccinated. There are exemptions from vaccination, in every state. Legally there must be exemptions; otherwise every case of vaccine injury would have an open and shut case. It's simple liability, and exemptions are their loophole.

There are **3 types of exemptions**:

1.   All states have a **medical exemption**. You must find a doctor who will write a note saying that your child is in danger from vaccines. That signature will be sufficient for lifetime exemption from vaccination.

2. **Religious exemption**. Several states have religious exemption from vaccination. Some require proof of membership in a formal religion. Others don't require that you specify.

3. **Philosophical exemption**. About 15 states presently offer this type of exemption. You just have to sign a waiver stating that you

have some unspecified philosophical objection to vaccination, and the kid is off the hook.

For some states, like California, the exemption form is printed on the other side of the immunization records form, and often they deliberately make copies of just the front side. So you have to know about it to ask for it.

People always say, "But they told me they won't let my child into school without his shots." Funny thing – even though required by law, it's almost unheard of for the school bean-counters to inform parents about exemptions, available in every state. You must know about your state's exemption form before you go in. Then all you have to do is present it. In most cases, once they see that someone is informed, they back down.

Why is this system of lying by omission in place? **$50 billion.**

EXEMPTION LAWS FOR ALL 50 STATES

Information about individual state exemptions from vaccines can be found at the government health office in the state capital, or at these websites:

  http://www.vaccinesafety.edu/cc-exem.htm
  http://www.ncsl.org/Default.aspx?TabId=14376

AFFIDAVIT OF EXEMPTION

There are now many other situations besides grade school and high school where vaccines are being arbitrarily required:

- colleges
- government jobs
- day care centers
- health care workers
- private businesses

to name just a few. Usually notification is simply given that vaccination is required, period. As we saw above, information on exemption is rarely offered. If just declining the shot doesn't work, there is another way out that is successful most of the time, by following these simple steps:

1. Type "Affidavit of Exemption" on a sheet of paper
2. Then type: "I hereby claim exemption to vaccinations because they may be harmful to my health or damaging to my immune system."
3. Go to a notary. Sign and date affidavit. Make copies.
4. Send a copy to the entity requiring the shots.
5. Send original by certified mail to the Legal Department of the entity requiring the shots
6. Keep your copy

To oppose your affidavit will now require a response, taking some action. Most will just let it slide; it will be the end of it. Those who would oppose you may miss the concept that by forcing you to undergo a medical procedure which you have already informed them may be harmful - this places liability for any adverse reaction on them. Putting it in writing would provide you with *prima facie* evidence that they are liable for any injury you might incur. A bureaucrat might miss this subtlety, but the legal department won't. Try it - it works.

With the recent vaccine fever and all the new untried vaccines appearing on the schedule, never before have the exemption forms been so important. Today, even parents who believe in vaccines are well advised to sign the exemption form, because then they can select the ones they want, instead of just leaving it up to this week's politics. Exemption forms put the power to choose back where it belongs : with the parent.

INDECENT PROPOSALS

Consider the 'workshop' held in Philadelphia in 2007 in which Paul Offit and others in the regulatory and vaccine manufacturing community proposed ways and means to end legal exemptions to vaccines, now available in almost every state. Other suggestions: public proscriptions of the unvaccinated, steps for criminal prosecution of the unvaccinated, eliminating the unvaccinated from hospital care and health insurance coverage.

Although these may seem like draconian measures unlikely to be put into effect on a nationwide basis any time soon, just the fact that they are being seriously discussed by the some of the top people in the vaccine industry should shock us into some kind of reality check about how serious these people are and the extent to which they are prepared to go in trying to force their experimental manmade versions of real or imagined pathogens into the bloodstream of our infants.

LEGAL DISASTER IN WASHINGTON STATE

There is a concerted agenda these days to replace parents' rights with government enforcement. Case in point: the 2011 legal catastrophe in Washington state, where the governor just rammed a bill through the state legislature that has eliminated the philosophical exemption. The real issue wasn't even the debate over whether or not vaccines are safe. Rather, it was a constitutional right that the citizens of Washington just lost, and most of them are happy about it!

Ever since vaccines have been mandated in the US it is the parents who have always had the individual right to decide whether or not their child will participate. It takes months of agonizing research in most cases to de-program oneself of a lifetime of conditioning, and then a modest amount of moral fibre to actually take the initiative to sign the exemption paper and free up the child's formative immune system from being an experimental petri dish for whatever neurotoxins the FDA decides to mandate that year.

And now people want to say – no, parents don't have that right. It is the government who should have total jurisdiction over the bloodstream of its citizens. Even though vaccine decisions are made by bureaucrats, not doctors. This is not a dramatization, but an accurate account of what just took place in WA state. [4] Sailing through with such little opposition, it is likely other states will follow suit in the near future. Remember this prediction.

WHO PAYS FOR NEW VACCINES?

With federal grant programs from NIH, the majority of the $100-$300 million price tags for "researching" a new vaccine and bringing it to market are siphoned out of the public trough. That's right: the fed pays beaucoup dollars to develop endless new vaccines that will be tested on live American children.

So let's recap the US vaccine situation:

1. Manufacturers don't risk their own capital in researching new vaccines; they receive NIH grants
2. If a vaccine is approved, the manufacturer gets the patent and reaps profits of $1 billion/year or more
3. No manufacturer is liable for vaccine deaths or injuries
4. The approval body - The FDA Advisory Committee - ACIP – is made up entirely of drug industry personnel

A dream come true, it took years for this system to devolve to its present mutation, but it is now entrenched into an unassailable position: a triumph of collusion between government bureaucracy, corporate manufacture, and legal status. Science comes in a poor fourth.

TRAVEL VACCINES

Another great marketing tool. The hook here is you're leaving the country for parts unknown. So that must mean unknown bugs for which you have no immunity, right? Wrong. Now of course we can't overlook the reality of little travel extras like amoebic dysentery, jungle rot, or Montezuma's revenge. It's just that fear of the unknown is a great opportunity for the vaccine sales force to violate your bloodstream by convincing you to put aside common sense in favor of the Magic Bullet *du jour*. Again, is there a separate industry involved in making travel vaccines, distinct from the dog and pony show outlined in the last hundred pages? Nope. Same guys.

When you travel you are going to be exposing yourself to a new environment – new stressors, new food, new gut flora, new air quality. So your immune reserves are going to be challenged as they try to keep your systems in equilibrium. At the one time you need it most why on earth would you want to handicap that immune system with experimental vaccines, loaded with manmade pathogens and additives? Common sense is all that protects travelers from disease, not vaccines. Care about food, drinking water, local plants, air, environment, supporting the immune system – these are the only defenses that ever protect anyone, home or abroad. For the last time, germs are the evidence of disease, not the cause of disease. Scavengers, not predators.

ANIMAL VACCINES

Love your dog, cat, or horse? Do you blindly subject them to every new vaccination that comes along? After reading this book, could you imagine there's an entire separate vertical integration of research, sales, marketing, and politics involved with the preparation and sales of **animal vaccines**? And that this industry has totally loftier ethics from that of the human vaccine cartels?

Big surprise - it's the same game, top to bottom. New research coming from Purdue University [17, O'Driscoll] found out that vaccines cause auto-immune response in dogs. In other words, vaccines are creating antibodies to the dogs' own DNA, as well as to their own collagen. Read the study!

This chapter is getting too long to go into it, but the reader is directed to the predictably horrifying *How To Protect Your Dog From a Vaccine* [331] as well as Dr Mason's *They Shoot Horses.* [332]

A LITTLE RESEARCH PROJECT

Find someone whose kids were never vaccinated. I don't know, just do it. Now ask if their kids get colds, allergies, infections, asthma... Just ask them. Ask them how their children's health compares to other kids. Try 10, 20, 30. Right, anecdotal. [293]

WORST CASE SCENARIO

When estimating the number of adverse vaccine reactions that get reported, most FDA and CDC sources use 10% as an estimate. (NVIC [261, 81]) FDA Commissioner David Kessler actually stated in *JAMA* that the actual number was closer to 1%! [310] But since the real number was **0%** before 1991, and since no studies have ever been done to verify the 1-10% figure, no one really knows. Seems like it might be a good idea to propose a worst case scenario, just to get a realistic feel for what the situation might actually be.

Let's say the 10% figure is really 5% or even 1%. No one can say that's impossible, because it's never been documented. In fact, in 1998 the NVIC did a survey of New York pediatric offices and found out that "only **1 doctor in 40** reports a death or an injury following vaccination." (DPT Vaccine Reports) [222] This means that in those areas **97.5%** of deaths from vaccines don't get reported. That could be the true nationwide figure.

So what if 97% of all adverse reactions to vaccines are never reported? Remember, vaccines can carry a slow virus which can hide out for years somewhere in the body. So maybe many of these adverse reactions haven't even shown up yet.

Maybe someone who gets a disease in 2010, cause unknown, is

really having a reaction to a vaccine given in the 1980s. And maybe this is happening on a mass scale.

Looking at the epidemic incidence of both degenerative and infectious disease in this country, it seems all out of proportion to our medical budget. Why? Drug shortage? Vaccine shortage? Hardly. Our downward spiral of health could be largely due to vaccine reactions and we wouldn't even know it. Who would tell us? The newspapers and magazines? The doctors chalked up to vaccine reactions. But the point is, **it's possible**. At the very least, vaccine reactions are a prime suspect in the recent increases in the following conditions:

heart disease	allergies	digestive disease
arthritis	apnea	tuberculosis
AIDS	asthma	autoimmune diseases
cancer	diabetes	nerve disorders
thyroid disease	chronic fatigue	poor vision
infertility	autism	learning disorders

The skyrocketing of all these diseases never happened until we started down the road of runaway vaccination.

Grim outlook? Sure. Just trying to figure out why we're so sick. Just look around – are kids healthier or sicker today than they were 20 years ago? Smarter or dumber? More or less inhalers in school? Mark Lappe talks about natural selection, survival of the fittest, and how vaccines have produced an artificial detour in our ability to evolve as a race, to refine our DNA. If that's true, the long-term survivors will be

the unvaccinated
those who are immune to vaccines   [290]

NEW VACCINES IN THE BULLPEN

Since the time of Pasteur and Jenner, the sale of vaccines has been the real motherlode for the pharmaceutical cartels. With the absurd Offit article [150] proclaiming that babies could handle 10,000 vaccines at a time, dozens of new vaccines are now in development. The focus is on the brass ring: APPROVAL. Besides AIDS vaccine discussed above, here are a few others in pre-game warm-up:

Cytomegalovirus	*Chlamydia*	**tobacco addiction**
Hepatitis C	**obesity**	**AIDS**
Herpes simplex II	**gonorrhea**	**pneumonia**
asthma	**dengue**	**longevity**
Respiratory Syncytial Virus		[98] [284]

Malaria, TB, meningitis, Alzheimer's, allergies, hay fever, diabetes, and tonsillitis vaccines are also in the pipeline. These vaccines are not theories. Hundreds of millions have already been spent on their "development." We will be seeing them shortly. [39]

FORM IS EVERYTHING

If FDA approval is more a matter of politics than science, then the drug cartels want to be ready for any eventuality. They know that vaccines don't have to work; in fact the diseases don't even have to exist. All that is necessary is the **presentation** of a threat and the presentation of a cure. This can be handled with control of medical studies and publications, popular press, FDA board members, and

Congress. [260] It's certainly not a conspiracy. This is just the way the world works.

The above list of vaccine hopefuls is alive. Two years from now there will probably be 50 new bugs that drug companies will be "developing a vaccine" for. This is the legacy of Pasteurian dogma – the Germ Theory. We have identified thousands of bacteria, viruses, and microbes. For modern medicine, theoretically they're all candidates for vaccine development.

> "We don't need to be finding vaccines for every organism
> out there."   - Stephanie Cave, MD   [185]

DARWINISM AND VACCINES

Are people becoming more or less aware of vaccine problems?

With the tens of millions spent annually to advertise and promote vaccines, it would seem that all parents would be absolutely sold by now. They're not. The percentage of **unvaccinated** children in the US is increasing very slightly every year, despite:

    incessant media endorsement
    school requirements
    the course of least resistance

The increase is astounding when one considers that to resist vaccination requires self-education - enormous personal effort, following up the spark of a new perception that hey, there might really be something to all this noise about vaccines, and I as a parent will do whatever is necessary to protect my child. Even if it means actually reading something. The struggle to step off the common treadmill thus becomes a war of attrition. A brick by brick proposition. A true awareness of vaccines can never be mainstream – not with the never-ending attacks on self reliance, self education, and allowing the child's natural immune system to develop unmodified.

The point of view expressed in this book can never be endorsed in popular media. It can never be the prevailing conventional outlook on vaccines, no matter how many children are damaged. Vaccines are here to stay. The majority of the children in the US will always be vaccinated. And the amount of vaccine damage will continue to increase.

Any upside to this dismal landscape? Well, the human species is subject to the same laws of **natural selection** as all other life on earth. Those with the weakest immune systems drop out. The immuno-suppressive effect of the immense viral load being forced onto the young through vaccines over long periods of time will certainly cause their line to have the least chance of replication of a viable progeny. It will dilute their DNA forever. In the US during the past 50 years, where the vaccine load has been increased by more than **2500%**, look at what is already clearly observable in the health and intelligence of our children: fatter, sicker, dumber. Play that pattern forward another 50 years, 100, 200. Nature will always take its course.

Anyone who studies the social and epistemological dynamics of the vaccine issue for enough time will eventually be confronted with the ultimate fruitlessness of direct confrontation on this issue, for the most part. The uneducated, and the militantly uneducated will always, always vaccinate their children. And thereby over time may be selected out of the species. It's neither good nor bad: it's simple genetics.

The survival of the Correctly Informed.

MESSAGE FROM THE PAST

To those who would leave the decision about whether or not to vaccinate up to their doctor, because it's too scientific and technical for the layman to understand, Dr Hadwen speaks from the past:

"the very moment you take a medical prescription and you incorporate it in an Act of Parliament, and you enforce it against the wills and consciences of intelligent people by fines and imprisonments, it passes beyond the confines of a purely medical question. .becomes essentially a social and political one." [191]

Still rings true today, a century later. The whole vaccine question is no longer just an issue of science, to be left to the "experts." Once politics and big money took over, anyone who takes the time to discover the source of funding behind the laws and clinical research and medical publication about vaccines in this country, anyone can get the Big Picture. One doesn't have to grasp all the scientific details of the immune system in order to make a decision about whether vaccines are dangerous or not.

Vaccines are not dangerous just because scientists don't know enough about the human immune system. They are dangerous because scientists don't know enough about the human immune system and yet vaccines are administered and required anyway.

SOMEWHERE MACHIAVELLI SMILES

Perhaps the darkest consequence of all the foregoing is that most of us have lost confidence in the inner curative power of Nature - the body's inborn wisdom. A hundred media snippets a day, week after week, year after year, have undermined our ability to even consider the notion that 99.9% of infants may be perfect as they are. Or that their pure blood is the most sacred medium in the universe, the crucible in which the human genome itself was meant to be safeguarded and passed on from age to age. Or that the immune system can only develop to its full potential if left to its own devices, largely unknown to human science.

Such natural, vital postulates as these sound foreign to our ears, even fanatical, cultist. Clear, rational, independent thinking has become so rare, so unwelcome, so feared in our world, where Conventional Wisdom on all topics of consequence is locked down tight, top to bottom. Adrift in this gallery of manufactured illusion, no effort is spared to keep one idea from surfacing: that we have all but lost the ability to trust our own instincts, to find the truth, and then to act on it.

CLARENCE DARROW

The appended reference list is just a cursory look at an immense body of literature that is at odds with current vaccination policies. If vaccinations are so safe and valuable, then why does the government have to pass laws to force people to get vaccines that aren't required in other free countries of the world, countries who have better health than we do? Why are there laws describing how people should be quarantined and deprived of property for refusing shots? Why were those parents in Maryland in 2007 forced to vaccinate at gunpoint?

Clarence Darrow, the famous lawyer at the beginning of the 20th century, asked: if vaccinations really work, then those vaccinated will be immune to disease, right? So what does it matter if some people choose to go unvaccinated? What do the vaccinated have to worry about? Aren't they protected?

The answer is obvious:: "It's the Money, Stupid!" (Null) [220]

UNAVOIDABLY UNSAFE

A new phrase entered the vaccine lexicon in a 2011 Supreme Court decision, which ruled that vaccines are **"unavoidably unsafe"** by their very nature. But instead of that being a sensible reason for exempting a child from vaccines, it was the closing argument the Supreme Court used to indemnify vaccine manufacturers, from now on – from being sued for deaths and injuries:

"In *Bruesewitz v. Wyeth* the Supreme Court ruled that Americans do not have a right to sue vaccine manufacturers for injuries that are the result of **defective design**. No other product is shielded from lawsuits based on design defects." [21]

How much clearer does it have to be? 68 vaccines are mandated for every child in this country. The Supreme Court says vaccines are dangerous by their very nature. And no parent can now sue the manufacturer if the child dies or is injured by the vaccine.

The Court is protecting the manufacturers here. So who is protecting the children?

When you were a child, who protected you? ❏

The school is public, not the child.
            -- B J Palmer

REFERENCES

1. AFP *Vancouver Sun*   Japan reports sixth infant death after vaccination   7 Mar 11
   www.vancouversun.com/health/Japan+reports+sixth+infant+death+after+vacci
      nation/4415756/story.html#ixzz1GF3n6RMj

2. England, C   Thousands of USA pregnant women miscarry after the H1N1 vaccine
   American Chronicle 4 Apr 2011   www.americanchronicle.com/articles/view/188385

3. Corderoy, A   Side effects worse than the disease   *Sydney Morning Herald*
      15 Apr 2011   www.smh.com.au/lifestyle/wellbeing/side-effects-worse-than-the-
                  disease-20100917-15gbm.html

4. Winkler, D   Health advocacy in the public interest   www.hapi.com   2011

5. Majewska, M   Vaccinated vs. Unvaccinated Children   *Age of Autism* 23 Feb 2011
            www.ageofautism.com/2011/02

6. Elber, G   Baby's injury spurs bill on vaccine   *The World*   19 Feb 2011.
         http://m.theworldlink.com/news/local/article_44a9c0e7-a115-553a-ae72-
   761f567f02f4.html

7. $260 M in vaccines trashed   *New York Post* p A8   2 Jul 2010

8. Centers for Disease Control   *Diphtheria*
       www.cdc.gov/vaccines/pubs/pinkbook/downloads/dip.pdf

9. Medical Economics   *Physicians Desk Reference*   2011.

10. Andrew Wakefield: lesson in ethics   www.thedoctorwithin.com   2011

11. Mann D   HPV shot prevents genital warts in boys   WebMD   2 Feb 2011.
      www.webmd.com/sexual-conditions/hpv-genital-warts/news/20110202/
            hpv-shot-prevents-genital-warts-in-boys-and-men

12. Kim, J   Weighing the benefits and costs of HPV vaccination in young men
       New England Journal of Medicine p 393   3 Feb 2011

13. Giuliano, A   Efficacy of quadrivalent HPV vaccine against HPV infection and
    disease in males   *NEJM*   p 401   3 Feb 2011.

14. Conflict of interest disclosure forms   *NEJM* for Kim ref [12] above
    www.nejm.org/doi/suppl/10.1056/NEJMoa0909537/suppl_file/nejmoa0909537_
    disclosures.pdf   3 Feb 2011.

15. Yazbak, E, MD
         Thimerosal Containing Vaccines, Part III   5 Apr 2011.

16. Fraser, H   *The Peanut Allergy Epidemic*   Skyhorse   2011

17. O'Driscoll C   The Purdue Vaccination Studies and Auto-antibodies   April 26, 2011.

18. Deth, R PhD   Chilling impact on vaccine-autism research   January 10, 2011.

19. Court Protects Vaccine Manufacturers, Not Injured Children
              US Newswire New York   February 22, 2011.
    http://newsystocks.com/news/3971363/court-protects-vaccine-manufacturers-not
    -injured-children
20. WorldFactBook   Central Intelligence Agency website www.cia.gov   2011.

21. Cornell Law School   SUPREME COURT OF THE UNITED STATES   22 Feb 2011.
     BRUESEWITZ ET AL. *v* . WYETH LLC, FKA WYETH, INC., et al.
              http://www.law.cornell.edu/supct/html/09-152.ZS.html

22. Aaby, P The introduction of diphtheria-tetanus-pertussis vaccine and child
              mortality in rural Guinea-Bissau: an observational study. *Int J Epidemiol.* 2004
              Apr;33(2):374-80. PMID: 15082643 [PubMed

23. Dr Julie Geberding named president of Merck   finchannel.com 8 Jan 2010.
24. Norwegian MP demands an answer from WHO:
         the country's biggest medical scandal theflucase.com *Nettavisen*   7 Jan 2010.

25. Taylor, L   EU to probe pharma over false pandemic   *PharmaTimes*   4 Jan 2010.

26. Child, Adolescent and Adult Immunization Schedule www.cdc.gov   2010.

27. Falco, M 2009 H1N1 flu strain will be in next season flu vaccine *CNN* 22 Feb 2010.
28. Paddock C PhD Swine flu false pandemic?   *MedicalNewsToday*   15 Jan 2010.
29. Olmstead D   www.ageofautism.com   2011.
30. Macrae F   The false pandemic: drug firms cash in on scare over swine flu
                                      The Daily Mail UK   18 Jan 2010.
31. O'Shea T   *The Last Resort*   thedoctorwithin.com   2011.
32. Wodarg W MD   Swine flu: they organized the panic   8 Jan 2010.
                              www.whale.to *L'Humanite*

33. Interview with W. Wodarg MD   www.wodarg.de/english/index.html
                                                              4 Feb 2010.
34. Bauerlein M   The dumbest generation   Tarcher/Penguin 2008.
35. National Vaccine Injury Compensation Program Statistics Report   2010.
           www.hrsa.gov/vaccinecompensation/statistics_report.htm
36. Hirschler, B   Bill Gates promises $10 billion for vaccines *Reuters* 29 Jan 10.
37. www.youtube.com   search *Bill Gates vaccines* TED conference   Feb 2010.

38. Shear, M   Obama declares flu emergency *Washington Post*   25 Oct 09.

39. Johnson L *Associated Press* Ailing drug manufacturers see growth 21 Nov 2009.

40. Barclay, L CDC issues interim guidelines   20 Oct 09.
           http://www.medscape.com/viewarticle/710977
41. O'Shea T   *The sanctity of human blood* 13th ed.   2009.
42. Salecky M   STATE OF WASHINGTON DEPT OF HEALTH OUTBREAK
    AND VACCINE SHORTAGE - SUSPENSION OF LIMITS   23 Sep 09.
43. Neergaard, L *Associated Press* –   Sep 21, 2009.
    http://news.yahoo.com/s/ap/20090921/ap_on_he_me/us_med_swine_flu
44. Cervical Cancer   Centers for Disease Control
                        http://www.cdc.gov/Features/dsCervicalCancer/

45. IARC Monographs, vol 90 *Human Papilloma Viruses* Lyon France WHO   2007
       http://monographs.iarc.fr/ENG/Monographs/vol90/mono90.pdf

46. National Institutes of Health   Early Results: 2009 H1N1 Influenza Vaccine
                    www.nih.gov/news/health/sep2009/niaid-21.htm
47. Sanofi Pasteur   http://clinicaltrials.gov/show/NCT00944073   Sep 2009
48. *Swine flu: global pandemic* and *Goodbye swine flu* www.thedoctorwithin.com 2009.

49. National Center on Shaken Baby Syndrome
     http://dontshake.org/sbs.php?topNavID=8&subNavID=41&navID=384
50. Autism Detox Program   www.thedoctorwithin.com   2011.

51. Kugler, S (AP) Officials say US deaths expected from swine flu   28 Apr 09
52. O'Shea T   *Avian flu the pandemic that can never be*   www.thedoctorwithin.com
53. Roan, S Swine flu debacle is recalled *Los Angeles Times* 27 Apr 09
54. Hunt M   Virology – chapter 13 influenza virus   U of S. Carolina
                        http://pathmicro.med.sc.edu/mhunt/flu.htm
55. CDC website   www.cdc.gov   2011
56. Autism Detox Protocol www.thedoctorwithin.com/autism/autism-detox-protocol/
57. *The Guardian*: World Health Organization   Margaret Chan   16 Jul 09
58. W.H.O. Health Advisory, April 2009, accessed in Swine-flu-vaccine.info/.

59. Engdahl FW   WHO 'Mr Flu' under investigation for gross conflict of interest   8 Dec 09

60. Voller,L   *Stærk lobbyisme bag WHO-beslutning om massevaccination* ,
      Google: Information.dk/215355.   Copenhagen, 15 November 2009

61. Interview with Epidemiologist Tom Jefferson MD:
            'A Whole Industry Is Waiting For A Pandemic' *Der Spiegel,* 21 July 2009

62. Stein, R   Flu Pandemic Could Be Mild   *Washington Post*   8 Dec 2009.

63. S. Attkisson - Swine Flu Cases Overestimated? CBS News Exclusive:
            H1N1 Not As Prevalent As Feared   Oct. 21, 2009.

64. Drummond, J   Missouri Health Advisory 22 Dec 08 CDC Issues Interim
    Recommendations for the Use of Influenza Antiviral Medications among Circulating
    Influenza A (H1N1) Viruses 2008-09 Influenza Season

65. Current Flu Season Worst in 4 Years - CDC says *Journal of Chinese Medicine*
            http://www.cjmed.net/news/   18 Nov 2008.

66.   McKenna M   Plant cancellation shows problems in flu vaccine business
  www.cidrap.umn.edu/cidrap/content/influenza/biz-plan/news/oct0308solvay.html
                                  Oct 3, 2008.

67. INFLUENZA PANDEMIC   United States Government Accountability Office
           Report to Congressional Requesters   September 2008.
      www.gao.gov/new.items/d08671.pdf

68. Grady, D   Study links hepatitis B and cancer of pancreas
              New York Times   1 Oct 2008.

69. Hassan, M   Association between hepatitis B virus and pancreatic cancer
      Journal of Clinical Oncology   vol 26 no 28 p 44557   1 Oct 2008.

70. Marks, J MD   The Relationship of Chronic Viral Hepatitis, Alcoholism, and
      Cirrhosis to Liver Cancer   www.medicinenet.com   22 Nov 2008.

71. FDA paper: Thimerosal in Vaccines   14 Mar 2008.
             www.fda.gov/CBER/vaccine/thimerosal.htm#1

72. Borka, A.   Polio up in Pakistan   *Reuters*   19 Sep 2008.

73. B Taylor ASTHMA Body mass index and asthma severity in the
         National Asthma Survey *Thorax* 2008; 63: 14-20; BMJ Publishing   2008.

74. Turner, J Esq lecture Protect Medical Freedom conference Washington DC 20 Jun 01

75.   Medical Economics   *Physicians Desk Reference*   2008, 2010

76. Chronic Conditions in Children Will Pose Future Health Challenges Investigators
    describe probable causes   Harvard School of Public Health   June 26, 2007.

77. Gallup & Yazbak,   When 1 in 150 is really 1 in 67   vaproject.org Oct 2007.

78. Peterson, L   Vaccine order upsets some, but Perry stands firm
                Associated Press   February 6, 2007.

79. Lopes, G   Vaccine center issues warning *WASHINGTON TIMES* Feb 3, 2007.

80. Smitherman L   Drug firm pushes vaccine mandate: Merck lobbies on HPV
                   Baltimore Sun   January 29, 2007.

81. National Vaccine Injury Compensation website   2007.
    www.hrsa.gov/vaccinecompensation/statistics_report.htm#claims_filed
    www.hrsa.gov/vaccinecompensation/statistics_report.htm#post_1988
82. Looney C   Intracranial Hemorrhage in asymptomatic neonates
                                    Radiology vol242 #2 p 535 Feb 2007.
83. McNeil, D   Africa: W.H.O. Approves Rotavirus Vaccine
                                    New York Times 13 Feb 2007.
84. Bridges, A   FDA: Rotavirus Vaccine May Harm Infants
              Associated Press   February 13, 2007.
85. US Dept of Education Facts from NLTS2
            http://ies.ed.gov/ncser/pubs/20073005/index.asp   2007
86. Foggo, D *Sunday Times*. UK Mystery illness paralyses girl given cervical cancer jab
    www.timesonline.co.uk/tol/life_and_style/health/article5337885.ece 14 Dec 2008.

87. Vesikari, T MD et al. Safety and Efficacy of a Pentavalent Human– Bovine
    Reassortant Rotavirus Vaccine *New England Journal of Medicine*
                                    vol 34 p 23   5 Jan 2006.
88. Colgrove, J Ph.D. The Ethics and Politics of Compulsory HPV Vaccination
              New England Journal of Medicine Volume 355: p 2389-2391 December 7, 2006.
89. Pringle, E   Lawmakers sever ties between CDC and Big Pharma
                                    Lawyers and Settlements August 21, 2006.
90. World Health Organization   Injection Safety - Fact Sheet #231
                        www.who.int/mediacentre/factsheets/fs231/en/ Oct 2006.
91. Children and Youth with Disabilities   National Center for Ed. Statistics
                http://nces.ed.gov/programs/coe/indicator_cwd.asp
            National Survey of Children Health Care Needs 11 Nov 08 http://cshcndata.org
92. National Center for Learning Disabilities   ncld.org home page

93. *MMWR*   April 7, 2006 / 55(13);371 Autism Awareness Month ---
                        www.cdc.gov/mmwR/preview/mmwrhtml/mm5513a8.htm
94. Infant Mortality: UNICEF UNDER-FIVE MORTALITY RANKING .
                                www.unicef.org/sowc08/statistics/tables.php
95. Tuerkheimer D   The Next Innocence Project: Shaken Baby Syndrome and the
            Criminal Courts   87 WASH. U. L. REV. 1   2009.
97. Alphavax www.alphavax.com   2005.
98. World Health Organization   Fact Sheet 289   Development of new vaccines
99. O'Shea T   *The post- antibiotic age*   www.thedoctorwithin.com

100. Kennedy, R F   *Deadly immunity*   20 Jun 2005.
                www.rollingstone.com/politics/story/_/id/7395411?rnd
101. Shahani, K PhD   Cultivate Health from Within   Vital Health 2005.
102. Ismail, A   Prescription for power – drugmakers lobbying ensures
                their legislative dominance   Center for Public Integrity   28 Apr 05.

103. Moskowitz, R MD   The Rôle of Vaccines in Chronic Disease
              American Journal of Homeopathic Medicine 98:15, Spring 2005.

104. Martin, WJ, MD   Interview   13 May 04   Burbank, CA
                            www.ccid.org/publications.htm
105. Geier, M Geier D *Review of the Relationship between Thimerosal and Autism*
            Institute of Medicine, US National Academy of Sciences, January 2004.
106. Anderson M The shaken baby debate...does this syndrome really exist?
       mediabistro.com/mka   **Discover**   **2 Dec 2008.**

107. CDC Vaccine Price List   www.cdc.gov   February 23, 2004.
108. Jefferson, T   Influenza vaccination: policy versus evidence
                              British Medical Journal   27 Oct 2006
109. O'Shea T   *HPV The first cancer vaccine*   www.thedoctorwithin.com
110. Immunization Safety Meeting 9: Vaccines and Autism   Institutes of Medicine,
          Washington DC   9 Feb 2004.   www.iom.edu/subpage.asp?id=18065

111. Akinbami LJ. The State of childhood asthma, United States, 1980–2005. Advance
data from vital and health statistics; no 381,: National Center for Health Statistics. 2006.

112. American Lung Association. Epidemiology & Statistics Unit, Research and Program
Services. Trends in Asthma Morbidity and Mortality, November 2007.

113. Bradstreet, Jeff MD   Presentation to the Vaccine Safety Committee
                of the Institute of Medicine,   February 9, 2004.
114. Bradstreet, Jeff MD   Virus Detected in Spinal Fluid of Children with Autism (c)ICDRC
            Melbourne F JUNE 9, 2004.   www.informedparent.co.uk/wakefield1.htm
115. Capell, K   Vaccinating The World's Poor *Business Week*   APRIL 26, 2004.
116. Haney, D   Flu shots unable to combat virus strain (AP) 17 Dec 03
117. CDC website: Diphtheria www.cdc.gov/mmwr/preview/mmwrhtml/mm5053a1.htm

118. Geier, M MD *Journal of American Physicians and Surgeons*   Spring 2003.
119. Manning, A Smallpox vaccination ceased *USA Today*   15 Oct 2003.
120. Olmstead D   Homeschooled   2005   theageofautism.com

122. Carbone, M MD Mesothelioma, SV40, environmental carcinogenesis
              Loyola U, Program in Molecular Biology   2003.
       www.meddean.luc.edu/lumen/DeptWebs/MolBio/html/carbon.htm
123.   CDC website   Pertussis   Outbeaks
             http://www.cdc.gov/pertussis/outbreaks.html   15 Mar 2011.
124. Yazbak, E MD   Regressive autism and MMR   2003.
125. *U.S. Newswire*   WASHINGTON, May 6, 2003. Smallpox: United States Allocates
              $100 Million for Smallpox Vaccinations

126. FDA: Summary for Basis of Approval (SBA) for Varicella Vaccine
                            www.fda.gov/cber/sba/varmer031795sba.pdf
127. Geier, M MD   Thimerosal in Childhood Vaccines,
            Journal of American Physicians and Surgeons   Vol 8 No 1   Spring 2003.
128. Smallpox: bringing a dead disease back to life 2004 www.thedoctorwithin.com
129. HR 4169 Mercury free vaccines act of 2004
                    www.govtrack.us/congress/bill.xpd?bill=h108-4169
131. Altman, L   Virus Proves Baffling, Turning Up in Only 40% of Lab's Test Cases
                                    New York Times   24 Apr 03.
132. Eli Lilly Material Safety Data Sheet on thimerosal 13 Jun 91.
        www.nationalautismassociation.org/pdf/thimerosalmsds.pdf
133. Haley, B PhD   http://whale.to/v/haley.html

135. US Dept of Education   Autism figures state by state 1993-2002-2007
                        http://www.IDEAdata.org/tables/ar_aa2.htm
136. King, W   Smallpox vaccine risky for others *Seattle Times* January 19, 2003.

138. Meckler, L, Associated Press WASHINGTON   March 27, 2003.
                    "Second worker dies of heart attack after smallpox vaccination"
139. *CBS News*   March 29, 2003.
                    Three heart-attack deaths cause delays in smallpox vaccination program

141. Burton, D   Congressional Hearing on Autism and Vaccines
                        House of Representatives C-SPAN   10 Dec 02.
142. Weldon, D MD   Congressional Hearing on Autism and Vaccines
                        House of Representatives C-SPAN   10 Dec 02.
143. Singh, V   Autism, vaccines and immune reactions
                        http://vacinfo.org/vijendra_singh.htm
144. Kew, O   *Science*   p356   Apr 2002.
145. Burton, D   Opening Statement - Committee on Government Reform:
                Vaccine Safety and Autism   June 19, 2002.
                www.house.gov/reform/020619_autism_opening_statement.html
146. Baskin, D MD Testimony to Congressional - Committee on
                Government Reform: Vaccine Safety and Autism   June 19, 2002.
147. Wakefield AJ, Montgomery, S *Measles mumps rubella vaccine:*
        Through a glass, darkly Department of Medicine, Royal Free and University
                College Medical School, UK   www.singlevaccines.com/wakefield2.htm
148. Polio cases roil debate   *Wall Street Journal*   16 Apr 2002.
149. Madsen, KM MD et al.   A Population-Based Study of Measles,
                Mumps, and Rubella Vaccination and Autism   *NEJM*   7 Nov 02.
150. Offit, P et al. Do vaccines overwhelm the immune system? Infants have the
        capacity to respond to an enormous number of antigens
                                    Pediatrics p.124   Jan 2002.

152. *Journal of Allergy and Clinical Immunology*   vol.110: pp357-365 2002.
153. Studies aim to improve pediatric end of life programs
                              Orange County Register   **p. 5   31 Jul 02.**
154. Williams, V WFAA-TV Dallas   19 Jun 02.
ww.wfaa.com/latestnews/stories/wfaa020619_am_thimerosalhearings.547d2350.html
155. Uhlmann, V Potential viral pathogenic mechanism for new variant
          inflammatory bowel disease. *Molecular Pathology* vol 55(2):84-90.   April 2002.
156. Frey, S et al. Clinical responses to undiluted and diluted smallpox vaccine
                    New England Journal of Medicine 3 64:17 p 11265   25 Apr 2002.
157. McRearden B   What Is Coming Through That Needle? The Problem of
                Pathogenic Vaccine Contamination   www.whale.to/a/needle.html
158. Reuters   Routine smallpox vaccine risky for eczema patients
                          www.reutershealth.com/en/index,html   10 Sept 2002.
159. Sylwester, R A Celebration of Neurons   p 17 ASCD   2002.
160. Drazen J MD   Smallpox and bioterrorism
                          New England Journal of Medicine 346:17 25 Apr 2002.
162. Jenner, E An enquiry into the causes and effects of variolae vaccinae
                SAV website: www.vivisection.info/article002.html   1798.
164. Davis, M Childhood Vaccine Purchase Costs in the Public Sector
                Vol 92, No.12   Am Journal of Pub Health   December 2002.
165. Acambis Says Early Smallpox Vaccine Results Encouraging   3 Sep 02.
            www.vaccinationnews.com/DailyNews/September2002/AcambisSays4.htm
166. Model Emergency Health Powers Act (MEHPA) Turns
                Governors into Dictators   http://www.aapsonline.org/   2002..
167. Beil, L Type of cancer, virus are linkedDallas Morning News   11 Mar 2002.
168. Jones, N Mutant polio vaccine regains virulence   *New Scientist*
            www.newscientist.com/news/news.jsp?id=ns99992047   14 Mar 2002.
169. Schuchat, A et al Bacterial Meningitis in the United States in   1995
          New England Journal of Medicine Volume 337:970-976 October 2, 1997
170. Horwin, M   PREVNAR A Critical Review of a New Childhood Vaccine
                          www.jabs.org.uk/forum/topic.asp?TOPIC_ID=75
171. U.S. Dept of Health and Human Services, Thimerosal to The National
            Toxicology Program, Safety Review Committee Meeting 3, 16 July 01
173. Bookchin & Schumacher The virus and the vaccine *Atlantic Monthly* Feb 2000.
                    www.theatlantic.com/issues/2000/02/002bookchin.htm
174. Kessler, D, MD   A Question of Intent   PublicAffairs/Perseus 2001.
175. Microsoft® Encarta® Online Encyclopedia 2001.
                        http://encarta.msn.com/find/Concise.asp?ti=049AB000
176. *The Columbia Encyclopedia*, Sixth Edition.   2001. Columbia University Press.
177. O'Shea, T   Smallpox: bringing a dead disease back to life 2004.
                        www.thedoctorwithin.com
178. *USA Today*   Asthma rates defy explanation   17 Aug 2001.
179. Goodwin, J   Vaccine? It's a question that is tearing families apart
                Redbook Sept 2000.   http://www.whale.to/m/sbs21.html

180. Bernard, S et al Autism: A Unique Type of Mercury Poisoning
                www.autism.com/ari/mercurylong.html ARC Research April 3, 2000

181. Hepatitis A: Creating a Market   www.thedoctorwithin.com
182. US Dept of Commerce --- Statistical Abstracts of the United States --
                                                - p 137 --- 2000.
183. NVIC Hepatitis B Reaction Report
                Townsend Letter for Doctors #205/206 p 148 Aug/Sep 2000.

185. Cave, S , MD lecture, DAN 2000 Conference San Diego   15 Sep 2000.
186. Koren, T *Childhood Immunizations*   Koren Publications   2004.
187. Borenstein, S Asthma At Epidemic Levels *San Jose Mercury News* 4 Sep 99
188. Dunbar, B PhD   *20/20* ABC Television Jan. 22, 1999.
189. Burton, D   *Congressional Hearing on Autism and Vaccines*
                                6 Apr 00, House of Representatives   www.c-span.org
190. Orient, J, MD   Statement of the Association of American Physicians &
                Surgeons to the House of Representatives   June 14, 1999.
                        http://perso.wanadoo.fr/bel/power/hepb2.htm
191. Hadwen, W MD The Fraud of Vaccination *Truth*   January 3, 1923.
                www.soilandhealth.org/02/0201hyglibcat/020119hadwin.toc.html
192. Hadwen, W MD   Sanitation Vs. Vaccination: the Origin of Smallpox
                                "Truth"   January 17, 1923.
193. Wallace, AR   VACCINATION A DELUSION - Its Penal Enforcement a Crime
                                London   1898.www.whale.to/vaccine/wallace/book.html
194. Rains, A J   Edward Jenner and Vaccination.
                                Priory Press Ltd.   p60 1974.
195. Arning, E *Vaccinations*   Encyclopedia Brittanica 9th edition 1889.
196. Hadwen W MD   The Case Against Vaccination   25 Jan 1896
        www.soilandhealth.org/02/0201hyglibcat/020119hadwin/020119
                hadwenrallytalk.html
197. Auwerter PG Changes within T cell receptor V beta subsets in infants following
                measles vaccination. *Clin Immunol Immunopathol.* 1996 May;79(2):163-70.

198. Halsey, N MD Limiting Infant Exposure to Thimerosal in Vaccines
                Journal of the American Medical Association (282) p 1763   1999.
199. James, W   Immunizations: The Reality Behind the Myth
                                Bergin & Garvey   1995.
200. Guyton & Hall Textbook of Medical Physiology Saunders   1996.
201. Burnet & White -   The Natural History of Infectious Disease
                                Cambridge U Press New York   1972.

202. Hume, E. Douglas   Bechamp or Pasteur?   Mokelumne   1923.
203. Moskowitz, R MD   The Case Against Immunizations
                                J Am Inst of Homeop p 21   Mar 1983.

204. Anderson, HB   The Facts Against Compulsory Immunization
                        Citizens Medical Reference Bureau   New York   1929.
205. Russell, PK, MD   Development of Vaccines to Meet Public Health Needs:
      Johns Hopkins University www.fplc.edu/risk/vol7/summer/russell.htm#top   1994.
206. US Dept of Comm. Historical Statistics of the U.S. Part 1Bureau of Census 1975
207. Sacher, R.A.   Widman's Clinical Interpretation of Laboratory Tests
                              - 10th Edition   F.A. Davis   1991.
208. Dorland, W.A.   *Medical Dictionary*   Saunders   1980.
209. Burton, Alec DO *British Medical Council* (272)   May 1950.
210. Murphy J - What Every Parent Should Know About Childhood Immunization
                              Earth Healing Products   Boston   1993.
211. McBean E   The Poisoned Needle   Mokelumne Hill   1993.
212. Strebel, P   et al - Epidemiology of Poliomyelitis in the U.S.
                              Clinical Infec Dis CDC p568   Feb 1992.
213. Alderson, M - International Mortality Statistics
                              Facts on File, Inc   ISBN 0-87196-514-3   1981.
214. Yiamouyiannis, J   Fluoride: The Aging Factor   Health Action Press   1993.
215. Neustaedter, R - The Vaccine Guide   North Atlantic Books   1996.
216. Colborn, T, PhD   Our Stolen Future   Plume   1997.
217. Bishop & Waldholz   *Genome*   Simon & Schuster   1990.

218. Snider, A -   Near Disaster with the Salk Vaccine. p40 *Science Digest* Dec 1963
219. Curtis, T   Possible Origin of AIDS. *Science* p 1259   29 May 1992.
220. Null, G - "Vaccines: Are They Really Safe" Part I, II, III, and IV
                              www.garynull.com/Documents/vaccines3
221. Hay, W. H. MD -   Address to Congress on the Lemky Bill
                              Congressional Record   25 Jun 1937.
222. NVIC DPT Vaccine Reports: Master List of Lot Numbers99   www.909shot.com
223. Garrett L -   The Coming Plague   Penguin 1994.
224. Baxby, D.   *History Today*.   March 1999.

225. Baron, J   *The Life of Edward Jenner* volume 2   London 1888.

227. Coulter & Fisher A Shot in the Dark   Avery   1991.
228. Toomey, J MD -   Reactions to Pertussis Vaccine.
          Journal of the American Medical Association vol.139 p448   12 Feb 1949.
229. Cody, C MD et al.   Adverse Reactions Associated with DPT Immunizations in
                              Infants and Children *Pediatrics* 68;5: p 650 5 Nov 1981.
230. Baraff, L MD -   Possible temporal association between diphtheria-tetanus
          toxoid-pertussis vaccination and sudden infant death syndrome
                              Pediatric Infectious Disease 2;1:7   Jan 1983.
231. Trollfors B Whooping cough in adults *BritishMedicalJournal* 12 Sep 81 vol 283 p696
232. CDC - Pertussis immunization: family history of convulsions and use of
                antipyretics *Morbidity and Mortality Weekly Report* 36:p 281   1987.

233. Shelton H   Save Your Baby: The Hygienic Care of Children 1993.
                                  www.whale.to/vaccines/shelton1.html
234. Madsen T - Vaccination Against Whooping Cough *JAMA* 101(3) p187   1933.
235. Stewart, G MD - Vaccination Against Whooping Cough: Efficiency Vs. Risks
                                                        Lancet Jan 1997
236. Kalb & Foote   Necessary shots? *Newsweek* p 75   13 Sep 99
237. Jensen, B, DC -   Empty Harvest   Avery Publishing   NY   1973.
238. Kendrick, P -   Use of alum-treated pertussis vaccine, and of alum-
        precipitated combined pertussis vaccine and diphtheria toxoid
                                  Am J of Pub Health vol.32: p. 615   1942.
239. Scheibner, V PhD   Vaccination: The Medical Assault on the Immune System
                                  Australian Print Group   1993.
240. Phillips, Alan -   *Dispelling Vaccination Myths*   5 Feb 1998.
                        www.unc.edu/~aphillip/www/vaccine/dvm1.htm
241. Mendelsohn R, MD   How To Raise A Healthy Child In Spite of Your Doctor
                                  Ballantine New York   1984.
242. Peltola, H et al. Hemophilus influenzae type b capsular polysaccharide
        vaccine in children: a double-blind field study of 100,000 vaccinees 3 months to 5
                        years of age in Finland *Pediatrics*   vol. 60 p. 730   1977.
243. Granoff, D et al. Hemophilus influenzae type b disease in children vaccinated
        with type b *New England Journal of Medicine* p. 1584 18 Dec 1988.
244. Medical Economics   *Physicians' Desk Reference*
                        1998, 2000, 2001, 2002, 2003, 2004, 2007, 2008
245. World Book, Inc.   *World Book Encyclopedia* p S-513   1994.
246. American Pediatrics Assn.   *Red Book* 1982 update in
                                  Pediatrics   vol. 70(5) p.819   1982.
247. Scheibner, V PhD Vaccinations: 100 Years of Orthodox Research   1993.
248. Horowitz, L   Emerging Viruses: AIDS and Ebola   Tetrahedron, Inc 1999.
249. Blaylock,R MD Excitotoxins: The Taste That Kills   Health Press   1997

260. Belkin M   Mindless Vaccination Bureaucracy   Belkin Limited
                        NYC   www.gulfwarvets.com/hep-b.htm
261. NVIC   Vaccine Reaction Reports Continue To Increase   Jun-Jul p 7   1994.
262. Chopra D MD   Quantum healing   Bantam 1989.
263. Dublin L,   *Health Progress, 1935-1945*, Metropolitan Life
                        Insurance Company, p 12.   1948.
264. Association of American Physicians & Surgeons DOCTORS CALL FOR
        MORATORIUM ON HEPATITIS B VACCINE -   aapsonline.org   8 July 1999.

265. Buynak E, PhD   Combined Live Measles, Mumps, and Rubella Virus Vaccines
                        JAMA (207) 12 p 2259   Mar 1969
266. Beers & Berkow, MD --- The Merck Manual ---Centennial Edition 1999.
267. NIH manual on hepatitis   www.nlm.nih.gov/medlineplus/druginfo/
        hepatitisavaccineinactivatedsy202902.html#Brands

268. American Academy of Pediatrics --- Policy Statement: Guidelines For Use
      Of Hepatitis A Vaccine   *Pediatrics* --vol 98 no 6   p 1207-1215 Dec 1996.

270. Salk, Jonas, MD --   quoted in *Science Abstracts* 4 Apr 1977.
271. Wakefield AJ, et al., Ileal-lymphoid-nodular hyperplasia, non-specific colitis,
      pervasive developmental disorder in children' *Lancet,* Vol. 351, 637-641 Feb 28, 1998.
272. Hadwen, W MD Verbatim report of an Address given at Goddard's Assembly
      Rooms, Gloucester, England January 25th, 1896   www.whale.to/v/hadwen.html
273. U.S. National Institutes of Health database on cowpox and smallpox
            www.ncbi.nlm.nih.gov/ICTVdb/Images/em_poxvi.htm
      www.ncbi.nlm.nih.gov/ICTVdb/Images/Fenner/poxb.htm
274. FDA Center for Evaluation and Biologics Research
                              Hepatitis Control Report, vol. 4, no. 21,   1999
275. *La Stampa* Albert Sabin quote   Torino Italia   8 Dec 1985
276. Sinclair, I   Vaccination: the hidden facts
                  www.vaccinationdebate.com www.whale.to/vaccines/sinclair.html
277. *Science* Division of Biologics Standards:
                  The Boat That Never Rocked   vol. 175, pp.1225-1230, 1972.
278. Carrel, A MD   Man the unknown   MacFadden   1935.
279. Hencke, H MD   The Germ Theory: A Deliberate Aberration   1995.
280. Hadwen, W MD   Microbes and War
281. Ruesch, H   Naked Empress   Civis   1992.
282. Gunn, T   Mass immunizations: a point in question p 14 1992
                  www.garynull.com
283. Koos BJ and Longo LD, Mercury toxicity in the pregnant woman, fetus, and
            newborn infant *American Journal of Obstetrics and Gynecology*
                              Oct 126(3):390-406   1976.
284. Bjune G, Gedde-Dahl TW Some problems related to risk-benefit assessments in
      clinical testing of new vaccines.   *IRB Rev Hum Subj Res*;15(1):1-5. 1993.
285. Bjune, G Effect of outer membrane vesicle vaccine of group B
                  meningococcal disease in Norway *Lancet* 338:8775, p1093 Nov 1991.
286. CDC *Morbidity and Mortality Weekly Report,*   4 Oct 1984.
287. Gardner, S Rising incidence of insulin dependent diabetes
                              British Medical Journal vol 315 p 713 1997.
288. Libman, I MD   Was there an epidemic of diabetes
                              Diabetes Care 21:8 p1278 Aug 1998.

290. Lappe, M   Breakout: the evolving threat of drug-resistant disease
                              Sierra Club Books, 1995.
291. Osterholm, M et al. Lack of efficacy of *H.* b polysaccharide vaccine
            Journal of the American Medical Association 260: p 1423 **1988.**
292. Scudamore J   the definitive vaccine website   www.whale.to   2011.
293. Parents of unvaccinated children   www.thedoctorwithin.com

294. Thyagarajan B, McCormick Characterization of homologous DNA recombination activity in normal and immortal mammalian cells. *Nucleic Acids Res* 1996 Oct 15;24(20):4084-91. PMID 8918816

295. Miller, G   Letters of Edward Jenner   Johns Hopkins   1983.

296. SAV website: www.vivisection.info/article002.html
    Smallpox critique: vaccination, eradication, animal experimentation

297. Gillis, J Pledge for smallpox vaccine *Washington Post*   3 Dec 2001.

298. Fudenberg, H MD Hazards of vaccines *J Clin Investigation.* vol 4 p 97-105 2000.

299. Susens, G MD   The FDA has failed us *San Francisco Medical Society* journal www.sfms.org/sfm/sfm301k.htm Mar 2001. www.whale.to/vaccines/kinsbourne.html

300. Christie C et al.   Resurgence of disease in a highly immunized population
    New England Journal of Medicine 331, no 1, p 16   7 Jul 1994.

301. The doors of perception   www.thedoctorwithin.com

302. Raspail, X, MD Raspail et Pasteur *Petit Journal*,   19 September 1888.

303. Vaccination articles and testimonies by medical doctors
    http://www.whale.to/vaccine/articles4.html

304. *Vital Statistics of the United States* 1937-1992

305. Burton, A, DO   Tetanus: one naturopath's view
    The Hygienist Autumn 1995 www.whale.to/a/burton4.html

306. Cave, S MD What your doctor may not tell you   Warner Books 2001.

307. *U.S. Newswire*   8 July 1999   aapsonline.org

308. Calling the Shots: Immunization Finance Policies and Practices   (2000)
    Institute of Medicine   National Academy of Sciences

309. EMD Chemicals, Inc   Thimerosal Material Safety Data Sheet
    www.setonresourcecenter.com/MSDS/EMD/DOCS/wcd00026/wcd026b4.pdf

310. Kessler, D MD   A new approach to reporting adverse effects
    Journal of the American Medical Assn vol.269, No.21, p.2785 2 Jun 1993

312. Blake, T Esq   SBSdefense.com

313. Traudt, J   The invisible world   http://healthandenergy.com/invisible_world.htm

314. Interview with Andrew Dodd , Esq vaccine injury attorney 2 Oct 02 310 316 6223

316. Thomas, S   Tetanus Vaccination *Journal of Inf Dis*   Nov 1927.

317. Benjamin, M   UPI Investigates: The vaccine conflict
    United Press International Investigations Editor   21 Jul 2003.

318. CDC fact sheet HPV Infectionwww.cdc.gov/std/HPV/STDFact-HPV.htm

319. Duesberg, P, Schwartz J Latent Viruses: No Evidence for Pathogenicity
    Progress in Nucleic Acid Research and Molecular Biology 43:135-204, 1992.

320. Benjamini E   Immunology: a Short Course   Wiley-Liss   2003.

321. Madsen, KM   Thimerosal and the occurrence of autism
            journal *Pediatrics* vol 112 no 3 p 604   Sept 2003

322. Langreth R   Booster shot *Forbes* magazine   12 Nov 2007.

323. Danish studies   www.whale.to/a/danish.html

324. Kogan MD *Parent reported prevalence of ASD* journ *Pediatrics* vol 124 5 Oct 2009
325. Schechter R MD   Continuing increases in autism
                        Arch Gen Psychiatry 65(1) p 94 2008.
326. Richet, Nobel lecture, acceptance speech, 11 Dec 1913
327. O'Shea T *Vaccination Is Not Immunization*   Immunition Ltd   2010
328. *New York Post* page A8.   2 July 2010.
329. video Dr Stan Burzynski   www.whale.to   2011.
330. Cauchon, D   FDA advisors tied to industry   *USA Today* p 1   25 Sep 2000.

331. Terifaj, P DVM   *How To Protect Your Dog From a Vaccine*
            www.dogsparesort.com/books.html

332. Mason C PhD They shoot horses but vaccinate dogs
                www.horsehealthmatters.co.uk/aboutus.htm

333. Students get leeway on whooping cough shots
                            Associated Press July 27, 2011.

334. Blaylock R MD   How the brain reacts to vaccinations   20 Jun 2010
www.youtube.com/watch?v=aUCCdCecLTo&feature=player_embedded&list=PLA77C01E
F916264F7

EPILOGUE

This is not an anti-vaccine textbook. This book is in favor of any vaccines that have been independently tested and found to be absolutely effective, with no chance of harm to the recipient.

It's not that vaccines don't work, or that vaccines don't do anything. Vaccines certainly do have an effect on the immune system. And they might temporarily delay the onset of some diseases. But why would we want to delay traditional, mild childhood diseases that have always been part of human immune development?

As for vaccine effects, these occur in a random, unpredictable, haphazard, inconsistent fashion. Vaccines simply do not do what they are said to do. Experimental as they are, loaded with toxic adjuvants and attenuated pathogens, the primary effect of vaccines on the immune system must be described as immunomodulatory or immuno-suppressive.

This has little to do with conferring immunity or improving the child's overall health.

Maybe you're asking how can doctors, drug companies, and the government allow a vaccine program to continue that is without a doubt killing children, causing permanent injuries, and offering no proof of effectiveness?

That is a much larger question. To have any hope of its being answered we have to somehow come to the realization, without hysteria or paranoia, through much study and research, of one unpleasant fact: man's enormous capacity for evil. And we have to confront some uncomfortable demons about human nature, the power of money, and the extent to which those in power will go in order to keep this river of gold flowing.

Jim Turner said it best: to force vaccines on an entire population of children when it is it known that some of them will be killed and some of them will be injured by doing so, but insisting that it's still good for the whole group is a bad moral policy.

Maybe, we human beings have a Higher self, a divine spark, the part of human nature that is generous and spiritual and altruistic and sympathetic to human suffering - the angel half of the strange species *homo sapiens*.

Unfortunately, the demonic half of human nature is just as real and just as powerful. And historically, benevolent leadership and humanitarian regimes have been the rare exception. Brute force, domination of the weak, intimidation, and the science of lying – these are what runs the powerful nations, and what fashions a people's value system – never more so than today. Turning away from identifying malevolence in the world just because it's unpleasant ultimately assures its triumph.

What do the purveyors of sickness and death look like? Monsters and devils, horror and darkness? Hardly. These people are often gracious, well spoken, with social aplomb. They have perfected the packaging of sickness, degeneration and death by wrapping it in hope, health, youth, and vitality. This well-crafted illusion is designed to steal our money, steal our time, burn away our precious life, and give us unnatural values.

What we seem to have forgotten today is that we don't need anyone's permission to live our lives, or instructions on how to live it. We still have the ability to do our own research and reach our own decisions, irrespective of mass media conditioning. This challenge is truly the final frontier. What lies in the balance could hardly be of greater import: the uninterrupted evolution of a child's immune system.

Going out on a limb a little here. Some readers may have noticed the look of the pure child during that first few weeks of life, when the infant looks at you with that "What are you?" – those big eyes. The parents are the first representatives of a species never before witnessed. The child so new, so innocent – still hearing the echoes of angels – is now suddenly cast into this alien place with these strange beings.

With an utter purity of spirit, so recently differentiated from the infinite pool: this is the unmodified natural child.

But it seems that parents of vaccinated children rarely understand the above, because they never got to observe it. In their child, that universal connection was rudely and abruptly severed by the full rush of a neurotoxic assault from vaccines.

After absorbing the research in this book, you may not feel quite so smug about ignoring your child's instinctive revulsion toward needles, turning a deaf ear to their screams, dismissing it with the mantra – for their own good. When is it ever a good idea to disregard our instincts?

Ultimately the defense of a child's bloodstream resides with the parent – protecting the child from the cold realities of the world, for a little while at least. Knowing what the reader now knows about the way in which decisions are made about how a vaccine gets mandated in children's bloodstreams - what can we reasonably expect from a body of legislators controlled by the biggest of the special interest lobbies? Do we rely on them for sound judgment about what is to be injected into that most delicate and sensitive medium in the universe – the formative human circulatory system?

Confronted with the above evidence about payoffs, deals, conflicts of interest rife within the regulatory agencies, do we really want to grant access to the bloodstream to such as these?

Real protection has to begin with information - sound information, not propaganda. And the information must come not only from those making their living selling vaccines.

Human health does not come from a drug or a vaccine or an insurance company. A healthy baby needs no outside assistance, no tampering with the blood. The mysteries of health lie within the body, not within the medical texts, or the writs of law.

Pure, uncontaminated human blood is indeed a sacred commodity. We will arrive at a position of profound gratitude when we finally come to appreciate the identity, the oneness, the nobility of an inviolate bloodstream. ❏